SIRTFOOD DIET

The Beginner's Complete Guide to Burn Fat and Lose Weight Fast with a 21-Day Meal Plan

By

Johanna Nicole Green

© **Copyright 2020 by Johanna Nicole Green**
_____

All rights reserved.

This document is geared towards providing exact and reliable information with regards to the topic and issue covered. The publication is sold with the idea that the publisher is not required to render accounting, officially permitted, or otherwise, qualified services. If advice is necessary, legal or professional, a practiced individual in the profession should be ordered.

- From a Declaration of Principles which was accepted and approved equally by a Committee of the American Bar Association and a Committee of Publishers and Associations.

In no way is it legal to reproduce, duplicate, or transmit any part of this document in either electronic means or in printed format. Recording of this publication is strictly prohibited and any storage of this document is not allowed unless with written permission from the publisher. All rights reserved.

The information provided herein is stated to be truthful and consistent, in that any liability, in terms of inattention or otherwise, by any usage or abuse of any policies, processes, or directions contained within is the solitary and utter responsibility of the recipient reader. Under no circumstances will any legal responsibility or blame be held against the publisher for any reparation, damages, or monetary loss due to the information herein, either directly or indirectly.

Respective authors own all copyrights not held by the publisher.

The information herein is offered for informational purposes solely and is universal as so. The presentation of the information is without contract or any type of guarantee assurance.

The trademarks that are used are without any consent, and the publication of the trademark is without permission or backing by the trademark owner. All trademarks and brands within this book are for clarifying purposes only and are the owned by the owners themselves, not affiliated with this document.

Table of Contents

Introduction 6

Chapter 1 The Importance of a Diet 9

    Why You Should Diet 13

    Blue Zones 16

Chapter 2 What are Sirtfoods? 19

    The Pilot Study 33

    Fighting Fat 35

    Muscle Maintenance 37

    The Science of the Sirtfood Diet 40

Chapter 3 The Sirtfood Diet Plan 43

Chapter 4 What happens after finishing the Sirtfood Diet? 56

    The Sirtfood Diet in Context 57

    How is the Sirtfood Diet Different from other Diets?... 59

    Sirtfoods and other Foods 61

Chapter 5 Pros and Cons of a Sirtfood Diet . 74

    Is The Sirtfood Diet For You? 75

    Frequently asked Questions 77

Chapter 6 Meal Plans and Recipes 83

Chapter 7 21 DAY MEAL-PLAN 187

Introduction

Millions of people spend years chasing every diet craze, every fad, crazy ideas and diet advice. The worst part about it is you'll probably end up right back where you started. The truth is most diets work but they also fail. When you set out on your diet journey, you may think that you're one and only goal is to lose fat, which in fact can be hard, easy or even in between. You'll probably succeed but the battle doesn't end, diet isn't just about losing weight, your diet should also be motived by health.

Ultimately, the key to losing weight is weighed by two choices. We can either decrease our calorie intake, or through exercise, increase calorie burn. Imagine a scenario in which you could skirt the dieting and instead enact a "skinny gene", without the requirement for intense calorie restrictions. If you were to enact these "skinny genes", a survival mode is triggered, where the normal growth processes and fat storage are ceased. What happens is that the body instead brings its attention to burning fat and activating genes that repair and rejuvenate our cells. The result is weight loss and an improved resistance to disease. How can you achieve this? By having red wine and chocolate.

The Sirtfood diet has become a favourite of quite a few celebrities in Europe and is most known for allowing the consumption of chocolate and red wine; mainstreamed by celebrities such as the popular Adele. It has been dubbed a fad by many and health experts are in fact questioning whether this diet is really credible and does it live up to its hype. However, according to its creators, sirtfoods are the secret to unlocking fat loss and disease prevention.

This is a diet rich in sirtfoods containing certain nutrients that are believed to be influential in the human body's capacity to burn off fat and boost metabolism. Founders of the Sirtfood Diet Aidan Goggins and Glen Matten conducted a pilot study in 2015, which yielded results of 39 participants losing an average of seven pounds in seven days. Sirtfoods are super foods, which when consumed activate our "skinny genes" similarly to that of calorie restriction. These genes are known as sirtuin.

You're probably wondering, does this diet even work? If you were to look at the diet's many celebrity endorsements; celebrities who have come forward and claimed that the diet has helped them to lose weight, build muscle and to look and feel great. Then yes the diet works, it works for celebrities who have dieting coaches and even personal trainers. So the might change your question to whether the Sirtfood Diet will work for someone like you? Well, there is only one way to answer that question. Continue reading.

Chapter 1
The Importance of a Diet

Nutrition is vital to our body and all of its systems to function properly. Good nutrition can help in healthy weight maintenance, reduced body fat, and provide the body with energy. According to the Foods Standard Agency, a balanced diet comprises of a variety of foods that are based on starchy foods and the consumption of at least five portions of fruit and vegetables per day. It is also recommended that you moderate the protein levels and having only small or occasional amounts of food high in fat or sugar.

About calories

The number of calories present in a food is a measurement of the amount of energy that is stored in that food. The average person needs to consume about 2000 calories every day to maintain weight. However, calorie intake can vary depending on age, gender and physical activity levels. Men in general need more calories than women likewise people who exercise need more calories than those who don't.

Foods are divided into groups, one of these groups being macronutrients. These are the main nutrients that make up the foods we eat and there are three, carbohydrates, protein, and fat. Most foods contain a mixture of more than just one macronutrient.

Carbohydrates

These are our bodies preferred source of energy. The body uses carbohydrtaes to make glucose, which is either immediately used stored in the liver and muscles as glycogen for later use. It is recommended that forty five to sixty five percent of your daily calories come from carbs. Carbohydrates are found in all plant sources, such as grains, vegetables, fruits, legumes and nuts, dairy, and foods that contain added sugars.

Measuring the effects of carbohydrates can help the management of glucose. The glycemic index is used to measure how quickly a food causes the blood sugar levels in the body to rise. The measure ranks food on a scale of zero to 100. Carb loaded foods with a high glycemic index are quickly digested and absorbed, causing a rapid rise in blood sugar has a high glycemic rating. High GI foods include

Glucose scores 100. A score of 55 or less is considered low, as in the following: honey, baked potatoes, white bread, white rice breakfast cereal, watermelon, instant oatmeal, pumpkins, rice cakes, crackers, bagels, cakes and doughnuts. Carbs that are low GI are broken down more slowly and cause a gradual rise in blood sugar levels; these are asparagus, broccoli, celery, cucumber, lettuce, peppers, spinach, tomatoes, chickpeas, cooked carrots, grapefruit, beans, pasta, nuts, apple, and croissants. Medium GI foods are white potatoes, mango, sweet potatoes, corn, couscous and spaghetti.

Protein

Mostly used in the body for building and repairing muscle and tissue. Proteins are continuously being broken down and replaced. The proteins in foods when consumed are digested into amino acids which are later used to replace the proteins in the body. Proteins take part in metabolic, transport, and hormone systems, making up the enzymes that regulate metabolism. They also protect the body from disease through its immune function.

It is recommended that ten to thirty five per cent of your calories come from protein. Protein is found in meat, poultry, fish, legumes (dried beans and peas), tofu and other soy products, eggs, nuts, seeds, mil and other dairy, grains and some fruits and vegetables. The proteins found in foods are called "essential amino acids," and they are histidine, isoleucine, leucine, lysine, methionine, phenylalanine, threonine, tryptophan, and valine.

Fat

Fats provide energy during exercise, in between meals, and in times of starvation. Fats aren't necessarily bad for you, but you only need a small amount. The recommended total daily intake of calories from fat is twenty to thirty five percent and less than ten percent should come from saturated fats.

Unsaturated fats are vegetables oils, salad dressings, avocados, ground flax seeds, nuts, seeds and fatty fish (salmon, sardines, and mackerel). Saturated fats are found in beef, pork, full fat dairy products, butter and several snack foods such as cookies, pastries and donuts. Trans fats are labelled as the extremely bad fats and are found in some margarines, deep fried foods, snack foods, such as chips and donuts.

Why You Should Diet

Diet planning is most often associated with short-term weight loss and restrictive food intake. However, a diet plan should be tailored to health status, steering your eating habits (what to eat, portions of what to eat, and when to eat), exercise and lifestyle management.

Starting a diet for weight loss and to improve health is a worthy goal, but can be quite overwhelming. There are bound to be some hiccups when starting something new as this means making a change. Before you decide on starting your diet journey, ensure that you are certain of your goal, why you want to achieve such and whether this will be for the better.

For many people, diet planning is about weight loss, better health and building their self-esteem. For others, it is about a health issue that they want to address or even a quick fix for example looking good for a special event. However, weight loss is most often the most desired of them all. There are many who feel pressured to lose weight; some persons begin dieting because they feel as though their weight is the cause of all their problems. While others suffer from poor body image or body dissatisfaction.

Body Mass Index (BMI), now the standard way of measuring body fat composition is calculated by dividing your weight in kilograms by your height in meters squared. It has now been declared that anyone with a BMI greater than twenty five is overweight and anyone with a BMI of less than thirty is obese. Given the great value placed on thinness, and the health risks that obesity poses, it is not that surprising that so many people continuously turn to mainstreamed diets in the efforts of losing weight. We are judged by society's standards of what being overweight is or not being thin enough. Given such, it is important to note your current weight before you decide on how much weight it is that would like to lose before beginning your diet.

Forget about looking good, forget about body image. What you put in your body is reflected by your health. Risk factors for chronic illnesses for example type II diabetes has been at an alarming increase as a result of unhealthy eating and weight gain according to the Centres for Disease Control and Prevention. It is recommended by the National Institute for Health, that persons with diabetes resort to a diet that is low in fat but also limit the intake of foods with added sugar and salt. Eating a healthful diet can help a diabetic person to lose weight if necessary, manage their blood sugar levels, keep their blood pressure and cholesterol within the target ranges and delay or even prevent complications of diabetes. Even with the recommended diet for diabetes, there are still many cases of persons developing diabetes. Similarly, in spite of blood pressure and cholesterol medicines availability, there is still continued increase in the death rate from cardiovascular diseases.

With that said the Sirt Diet is said to be quite beneficial when it comes on to these diseases. Persons living in the blue zones partake in a plant based diet consisting of kale, buckwheat and other herbs, which based on research, are loaded with sirtuin activating nutrients. It is believed that this diet along with exercise and social wellbeing are what contribute to them being healthier and less likely to develop chronic diseases. Overall, why is dieting important? The best answer is to better one's health.

Blue Zones

Though sirtfoods is a recent nutritional finding, it is evident that other cultures have been reaping their benefits for a long time. Benefits, that would include increasing muscle mass and weight control. There are five regions around the world where the population is known to live longer when compared to the west these are known as the Blue Zones. A concept developed by author and National Geographic Fellow Dan Buettner. They not only tend to live longer, but also have remarkably low rates of cancer, heart disease, diabetes and obesity.

They have a strikingly high concentration of persons living to be over 100 years old. These blue zones include Okinawa in Japan, Ogliastra Region in Sardinia, The Nicoya Peninsula in Costa Rica, the community of Seventh Day Adventists in Loma Linda in California and Ikaria in Greece. The food choices may vary from one region to the next but the blue zone diets are mainly plant based, with a ninety five percent of daily food intake stemming from fruits, vegetables, grains and legumes. Processed foods are typically avoided as well as meat, dairy, sugary foods and beverages.

These individuals follow a wholesome diet, this however, is not the only factor that leads to longevity, and they also have a high level of physical activity, low stress levels, strong social connections and a strong sense of belonging and purpose. Nevertheless, their robust but vibrant, nutrient filled eating habits appear to be the main factor in their exceptional health. Studies done on the blue zones show where the natives within these areas have a diet that is high in polyphenols. They indulge in leafy greens such as kale, and whole grains, dominating their meals all year long, which are sirtuin activating nutrients.

Olive oil isn't the only plant based oil but it is definitely one of the most often used in the blue zones. Studies show where consuming olive oil increase good cholesterol and lowers bad cholesterol. For middle-aged people in Ikaria, it was found that about six tablespoons of olive oil is used daily which seems to cut the risk of dying in half. Olive oil is one of the twenty sirtfoods that is included in the sirtfood diet.

Some other sirtfoods that make up the blue zone diet include coffee, Sardinians, Ikarians and Nicoyans all drink and abundant quantity of coffee. Research has associated coffee drinking with lower rates of dementia and Parkinson's disease. People in the blue zones, drink one to three small glasses of red wine per day, it is believed that people who drink red wine in moderation tend to outlive those who don't. Tea plays an important part in the blue zones diet. Okinawans for example, nurse green tea all day. It has been shown to lower the risk of heart disease, and several cancers. The Ikarians drink herbs such rosemary, wild sage and dandelion which are all known to reduce inflammation.

A number of studies have been conducted on the diet of those who live in the blue zones. These studies have shown that blue zone areas are home to some of the healthiest and longest living people in the world, eating a plant-based diet, drinking moderate amounts of alcohol, exercising and having a good spiritual family and social networks. However, it has been found that when those inside the blue zones migrate to the west, they develop the practices and culture and even the diseases. This shows that good health is influenced by our diet.

Chapter 2
What are Sirtfoods?

The Sirtfood Diet was created by nutritionists Aiden Goggins and Glen Matten. The diet imitates the effects of fasting and exercising. It pushes individuals toward other foods without focusing on the foods that should be taken out of one's diet. The Sirtfood Diet promotes the consumption of "sirtfoods" which are high in sirtuin.

The diet is centered around these sirtfoods, which are a group of everyday plant foods rich in sirtuin activators. They are protein types which activate the so called 'skinny gene' pathways in the body. These pathways are the exact same ones that are usually activated by fasting and exercise and have been shown to play a role in burning fat, increase muscle mass and overall improve health. In countries such as Japan and Italy persons have already included sirtfoods as a part of their traditional diet. Both these countries are usually ranked as the healthiest in the world.

Researchers conducted a study, exploring the link between dietary habits of more than 124,000 people and the changes in body weight over a twenty-four-year period which ended in 2016. It was found that consumption of certain plant foods in the American diet prevented weight gain, while others had no effect at all. This led to the consideration that consuming foods that are rich in certain types of natural plant chemicals called polyphenols are impactful in the prevention of gaining weight as we age. So, what does this mean? It means that not all plant foods are the same when it comes on to regulating weight. We should rather, look into plant foods high in polyphenol content and their capability of activating our "skinny genes".

The foods that we try to wean off of such as chocolate, coffee and tea are actually heavily dosed with sirtuin-activating polyphenols. The consumption of cocoa has now been proven to activate sirtuin genes with the many benefits of controlling weight through fat burn, improving muscle function and lowering appetite. Aidan and Goggin founders of the Sirtfood Diet have identified twenty foods that are rich in polyphenols which have been shown to activate the sirtuin genes.

So what are these magical 'sirtfoods'? They include matcha green tea, dark chocolate (85% cocoa), lovage, celery, parsley, turmeric, kale, garlic, capers, red wine, strawberries, red onions, soy, extra virgin olive oil, buckwheat, walnuts, medjool dates, rocket (arugula), bird's eye chilli, and coffee. Each of these foods has their own impressive health qualities, but nothing compares to when they are combined.

How about that? Losing seven pounds in seven days all while eating chocolate and drinking coffee and red wine. There haven't been any officially barred foods on the sirtfood diet as yet. Some of these foods you may already know while others are simply just new to you.

Capers

You might be asking what capers are. These are pickled flower buds which grow all over the Mediterranean, having only 23 calories per 100 grams and providing nutrients such as calcium, iron and potassium and serving as flavour enhancers and boosters. They are salty, dark green and pellet like and packed with sirtuin-activating nutrients. Once the caper buds turn into flowers they are pickled in vinegar or preserved in salt. They add a bright and briny taste to savoury dishes, for example they can be sprinkled over roasted cauliflower or a salad.

Celery

Celery from earliest times has been dubbed a medicinal plant, aiding in detox and cleansing to avert illness. The most nutritious parts are the hearts and leaves, especially if doing a shake. The bitter ones with a strong green colour are recommended. Celery contains apigenin and luteolin which are major sirtuin activating nutrients. It can be eaten as a snack or be used in salads and soups or as a garnish on certain dishes.

Buckwheat

Buckwheat has been around for centuries, mainly consumed by Asian and East European countries. It is now becoming increasingly popular in the western countries because of the many health benefits that it offers. Buckwheat, related to rhubarb is a fruit seed and its seeds are rich in carbohydrates, as such it is sometimes called pseudo cereal. Though it is not really a grain, it can be used like one in cooking and can be used as an alternative to rice, pasta and bulgur wheat.

Buckwheat is quite healthy, versatile and is naturally gluten free. It is also available in a number of different forms for example, buckwheat seeds, pasta, flour and noodles, it is best to use the wheat free version. Buckwheat often referred to as a superfood is contains the sirtuin-activator called rutin and is high in protein and fibre. It contains 66 calories for an 80 grams cooked portion, 40 grams when uncooked and practically no fat. Additionally, a diet comprising of buckwheat is linked to lowered risk of high cholesterol and high blood pressure and even weight loss as it reduces food cravings. Buckwheat can be used as a side dish for curry or stew.

Bird's Eye Chilli

This also referred to as Thai chillies and contains the major sirtuin-activating nutrients Luteolin and Myricetin. Chilli originated in the Americas and has been in the human diet from 7500 BC. There are more than 200 varieties, ranging in heat from mildly warm to extremely hot, but bird's eye chilli is greater in sirtuin activators than the milder ones used. It is known for its weight reducing qualities and can contribute to increased metabolism by increasing your temperature. A faster metabolic rate, along with proper digestion and waste expulsion, can aid in the reduction of fat build up.

Medjool dates

Medjool dates are a type of tree fruit originating from the Middle East and North Africa. They contain approximately 66 calories each and as such are a good alternative to other desserts with lots of calories. Medjool dates are usually dried naturally, by allowing them to ripen and then sun drying whilst they are still on the tree. They can be eaten as a snack alone, with crackers or mixed with yoghurt for breakfast serving as they are a good source of fibre and essential minerals, potassium, magnesium, copper and manganese.

Dark Chocolate (Cocoa)

The Kuna American Indians, in the San Blas Islands of Panama show exceptionally low rates of chronic diseases such as high blood pressure, obesity, diabetes, cancer and early death. The Kunas, main supply of fluid is a beverage that is made from cocoa that is locally grown. Rich in polyphenols called flavanols especially that of epicatechin, making it a Sirtfood.

For chocolate to be counted as a sirtfod it has to be 85% pure cocoa, which is needed for the sirtuin activation. The flavonol-rich kind is said to improve blood pressure, blood sugar control and reducing high cholesterol. It also strengthens the body's defense mechanisms and puts diseases at bay.

Coffee

Coffee can boost weight loss as it helps the body to burn fat faster through the stimulation of the nervous system. The nervous system in turn signals the fat cells to break the fat down. It is recommended that you drink it black as evidence show where milk can actually reduce the absorptions of sirtuin activating nutrients. The healthiest coffee would be that of the organic dark roast, grounded from fresh whole coffee beans. Studies have shown where coffee can protect against quite a number of health conditions such as cancer, type II diabetes and heart disease. It is advised that you do not consume more than five cups per day but one way to have a balance between the risks and benefits would be to drink between one to two cups in the morning and drinking the green tea in the afternoon.

Extra Virgin Olive Oil

In the Mediterranean, olive oil is often used in dishes. It was cited as a cure-all by Hippocrates and it is now confirmed by modern science to be of great health benefits. Olives in particular contain major sirtuin activating nutrients called oleuropein and hydroxytyrosol. These are antioxidant polyphenols, helping to keep plants healthy, hardy and resistant to disease which when eaten by us provide the same benefits. This type has more sirt benefits and a more satisfactory peppery taste. It is advised that only two tablespoons be used per day. According to chief oil maker Leandro Ravetti, a diet that is rich in extra virgin olive oil delivers a greater and longer lasting weight loss results than a diet that is low in fat.

Matcha Green Tea

The consumption of green tea started more than 4,700 years ago. It began with Chinese Emperor Shen Nung, producing a delightful and refreshing drink composing of green tea leaves. Green tea later became known for its medicinal and healing properties. The people of Asia are notable for their high consumption of green tea and it is for this reason that they have some of the lowest rates in terms of cardiovascular illnesses and lung cancer, especially in Japan.

Matcha has been in the Japanese culture dating back from the 12th century. It differs from regular green tea because of how the leaves are produced and is far less processed; it is kept under the shade as a way of preserving its natural nutrients. Matcha green tea is a bright green powder, stirred into warmed liquid. This is rich in antioxidants and cancer fighting compounds and is all around one of the best remedies out to date. Matcha green tea raises metabolism and also aids in weight management, its benefits have been backed by many scientific researches. Adding a slice of lemon increases the absorption of sirtuin-producing nutrients. Matcha can be enjoyed as a regular tea or be used in a green smoothie.

Green tea because of its thermogenic effect intensifies the amount of energy that the body burns resulting in fat loss and muscle maintenance. Green tea, when combined with a diet rich in leafy greens, soy, spices and herbs similarly to that of the Okinawa people provide the benefits of longevity and a healthier body.

Kale

Kale is referred to as a superfood. A cup of raw kale contains 2.4 grams of dietary fibre, which aids in reducing hunger and ultimately weight control. How? Instead of eating potato chips, try kale chips baked with garlic and black pepper. Kale is rich in vitamins, minerals and protein and also low in calories. In just a single serving, you can come close to getting your recommended daily allowance of anti-inflammatory vitamins A, C and K. It has a great amount of sirtuin activating nutrients called quercetin and kaempferol. Massage kale with olive oil and lemon juice and serve as a salad, or use as a base in your green juice.

Lovage

This is a herb that can be grown on a windowsill. It is rich in quercetin, an antioxidant that has multiple health benefits. Its taste is described as a cross between celery and parsley with a hint of curry and aniseed. Lovage can be used in many ways, for example as a garnish, in omelettes, in salads or even steamed as a side. It can also be used in your stir-fries.

Parsley

Parsley is an herb that is popularly used in American, Europe and Middle Eastern dishes. It is mostly used to enhance flavours for dishes such as salads and soups. Parsley is low in calories but rich in other nutrients such a vitamin A which aids in your immunity and is good for the skin. It also contains vitamin C which improves heart health and is a powerful antioxidant that protects against cell damage. Parsley can be used in a smoothie or juice, as a garnish on pastas, and pestos.

Red onion

Red onions contain twice as many antioxidants than any other onion as such they are vital in an anti-inflammatory diet and sirtfood lifestyle. They contain the major sirtuin-activating nutrient, quercetin and antioxidant anthocyanin which prevents the nitrification of dietary and cellular fatty acids. Ensure that you utilise the outer, fleshy edible parts as much as you can. It is sweet enough to be eaten raw and is a better variety. Can be chopped and added to a salad or be eaten within a burger.

Red wine

Contains major sirtuin-activating nutrients resveratrol and piceatannol, which is heat stable as such it is beneficial to cook with. It can decrease the chance of having a stroke, heart attack as well as cancer. According to over 84 studies on alcohol, drinking a small amount can lessen the overall risk of death from heart conditions by 15 to 25%. It has also been proven to to reduce the risk of several types of cancer as the phenolic compounds found in red wine prevent the initiation, progression and growth of cancer cells. One such wine would be Pinot noir which is rich in sirtuin nutrients.

Rocket

Arugula also known as rocket is a pungent green salad leaf with a distinctive peppery taste. It is very popular in the US food culture, coming from Mediterranean as the base of many dishes. Before it became a salad leaf, it was used by ancient Greeks and Romans for medicinal purposes. Rocket is high in the sirtuin-activating nutrient quercetin and kaempferol which are believed to be good for the skin. When paired with extra virgin olive oil, the two make a very strong sirtfood combination that can be the base for your salads.

Soy

Asian countries such as China, Japan, and Korea have always had soy products as a regular in their diet. It was found that countries that have a high soy diet, have markedly lower cancer rates, as soya beans contain polyphenols and also include the sirtuin activators formononetin and daidzein. Soy products are more beneficial when they are mainly natural such as tofu. Soybeans and miso are high in sirtuin activators and can be included in stir-fries.

Strawberries

Strawberries contain the sirtuin activator fisetin. Though sweet, strawberries only contain 1 teaspoon of sugar per 100 grams. Research suggests that they improve the body's capability to handle carbs that are rich in sugar.

Turmeric

This is a spice that has been in use for many years due to its healing properties. Turmeric contains curcumin which is a strong antioxidant, reducing inflammation in the body thus helping to prevent cancer, heart disease, and other various degenerative conditions. Often used in the traditional Indian cooking, turmeric is believed to play a significant role in the lowered cancer rates in India when compared to Western cultures. Besides it anticancer properties, turmeric also have be shown to have other sirtuin-activating health benefits. It also has another unique strain of curcumin, which can be absorbed more easily and has been shown to regulate cholesterol levels, reduce inflammation and improve the control blood glucose levels. Researchers have tapped into its mechanism of averting weight increase and treating obesity.

Cooking it in liquid and adding fat and black pepper better increases it absorption.

Walnuts

Walnuts are the oldest tree food, dating back to the 7000 BCE, originating from ancient Persia. It has been dubbed by the Nuval system as the healthiest nut of them all, though it is high in fat and calories. It is however, known for weight reduction and lessening the risk of metabolic diseases for example diabetes and heart disease due to sirtuin activation. Though high in fat and calories, it reduces metabolic disease. These can be smashed with parsley and used for sirt-flavoured pesto.

Garlic

With healing and rejuvenating properties, garlic has been considered a wonder food dating back to thousands of years ago. It is a natural antibiotic and antifungal, The nutrient allicin, found in garlic which gives it its aroma works together with the sirtuin-activating nutrients ajoene and myricetin.

The Pilot Study

A clinical trial was conducted testing the effectiveness of the sirtfood diet weight loss. The trial was conducted in a private fitness centre in Chelsea, London by the diet's creators Goggin and Matten. The study consisted of 40 participants, and the results included 39 of these participants losing seven pounds while maintaining and also increasing muscle tissue.

This fitness centre had its own restaurant, which was beneficial in that it provided the opportunity to not only outline the diet but also to bring the diet to life. Members for seven days in row followed the sirtfood diet plan and their progress tracked from the start to finish. Their weight and how their levels of fat and muscle changed were also monitored, along with the measuring of their metabolic processes. This was done to assess whether the diet had any effect at all on their blood glucose and blood fats levels.

For the first three days, calories were restricted to 1000 per day which was somewhat of a semi-fasting. In doing this, growth signals in the body were decreased and old debris swept from cells which enacts the burning of fat. The study boasted a high percentage of 97.7 percent in terms of adherence. The aim was to achieve the fat-burning effects of this calorie restriction through a heavily based sirtfood packed diet. This was successfully attained by having a daily diet of three sirtfood rich green juices and one sirtfood rich meal.

The final four days of the program involved an increase in calories to 1500 per day. This was enough to lessen growth signals and fat burning signals maximized. Certainly, the diet was filled with sirtfoods, with two sirtfood-rich green juices and two sirtfood-rich meals per day.

The diet was tested by forty members and ended with thirty-nine members completing the program. Twenty one of which were women and eighteen who were men. Two of the thirty nine were obese, fifteen were overweight and twenty two had a normal BMI. The results were consistent, with an average of seven pounds in weight loss, especially noticeable within the abdominal region, in seven days while considering muscle gain. Remarkably, persons also maintained muscle mass. An improvement in body composition was also observed in all participants. Participants also reported feeling and looking better and ultimately healthier.

Fighting Fat

The pilot study done on the Sirtfood Diet found that persons were losing weight without losing muscle and this weight loss was mostly fat loss. Generally speaking, fat reduction normally requires a lot of sacrifice where you either have to decrease your calorie intake or partake in vigorous exercise plans or even both. We can only truly appreciate the results of the pilot study, when we begin to understand what truly happens to fat cells when sirtuin activity is increased.

Lean Genes

The level of Sirt1 in humans has been found to be remarkably lower in person's body fat who are obese, when compared to persons who are at a healthier weight. Leaner people and those who have a harder time gaining weight have increased Sirt1 gene activity. We can then consider how important sirtuins are in ascertaining whether we gain weight or lose weight and why by increasing sirtuin activity is linked to weight loss and muscle gain results.

Fat Burning

Peroxisome proliferator-activated receptor-Y (PPAR-Y) which turns on the genes that are necessary for synthesizing and storing fat. The rapid increase of fat can be halted by cutting off the supply of PPAR-Y. How? Through Sirt1. Sirt1, puts a stop to the producing and storing of fat but also alters the metabolic processes so that our body begins to rid itself of the excess fat. The mitochondria aids in this whole fat loss process by increasing fat burning.

WAT or BAT

White adipose tissue is a type of fat that is related to weight gain. WAT is responsible fat storage and fatty acids being released when energy is required.

Brown adipose tissue transforms chemical energy into heat, which prevents obesity and other metabolic disorders.

Muscle Maintenance

In typical weight loss diets, people tend to lose both fat and muscle. In depriving the body of energy, cells go from growth mode to survival mode and use the protein from muscle as fuel. In losing fat and retaining or gaining muscle, you look leaner and toner. The more muscle mass you have the more energy is being burnt and this aids in further weight loss and increases the possibility of long term result. Sirtfoods, help to maintain muscle mass and burning more fat with only a slight drop in the metabolic rate.

Muscle mass is an indicator of well-being and healthy aging. Maintaining muscle mass diminishes the risk of developing chronic illnesses such as diabetes and osteoporosis and keeps us active into older age.

Sirtuins, in their method of maintaining muscle is beneficial in stress-related disorders, including depression.

Once Sirt1 is activated, muscle breakdown is eliminated. Sirtuins not only preserve muscle mass, they also work to intensify skeletal muscle mass. Muscles consists a unique type of stem cell called satellite cell, which controls muscle expansion and restoration. They are pulled into action when muscles are damaged or when under stress, this account for our muscles getting bigger during training or exercise. Sirt1 plays a key role in activating these satellite cells. Without Sirt1, muscle mass is reduced as they no longer possess the ability to grow or regenerate effectively. By increasing Sirt1 activity, we kick start the satellite cells, in turn promoting muscle growth and recovery.

We have two types of skeletal muscle, type I and type II. Type I is for activities that lasts longer, while type II is short spanned but intense activities. In terms of fasting, Sirt1 activity is only increased in type I muscle fibers while it decreases in type II. This means that during fasting, type I muscle fibers size is sustained and also increases while in type II, muscle begins to break down and generate energy as fat burning is slowed. Type II fibers are the chunk of our muscle definition, whilst we see a growth in type I fiber mass, we still experience a great loss of muscle when we engage in fasting. However, if you increase Sirt1 activity levels by partaking in a diet that is high in Sirtfoods, muscle loss is put at bay, this was evident in the pilot study done in 2015.

Like any other cell in the body, muscle does age and as it ages, there is a reduction in the capability of activating Sirt1. What this does is to decreases its responsiveness to exercise benefits and become more susceptible to injury from free radicals and inflammation, known as oxidative stress. If we are able to heighten Sirt1 activation, then we can put a stop to the aging and decline of muscles. In doing so, the health benefits would be endless, benefits such as stopped bone loss, the prevention of increased chronic systematic inflammation plus improvements on mobility and in general, the quality of life. As shown in research, older people with higher levels of polyphenol in their diet have greater defence against a decline in physical performance due to aging. To conclude, sirtuin activity levels are crucial to muscle growth, loss and function.

The Science of the Sirtfood Diet

The Sirtfood Diet has the ability to actuate certain genes that exist in our bodies. These genes are called sirtuins and there are seven different ones. Sirt1 is found in the cell's cytoplasm and Sirt3 in the mitochondria. They carryout multiple different functions but mainly eliminate acetyl groups from other proteins. Sirtuins is derived from Sirt, a group of Silent Information Regulator proteins that increase muscle efficacy, increase the metabolic process, amps the processes of burning fat, aids in the repairing damaged cells and reduces inflammation. In short, sirtuins make us healthier, fitter and leaner.

Sir2 was the first sirtuin to be uncovered in the 1970s, controlling fruit flies mating abilities. Similar proteins were discovered in the 1990s, with every organism having a different number of sirtuins. Yeast for example has five while a bacterium only has one. Humans have seven as was mentioned previously and with the experiments done on mice, they were found to have the same as humans. An interest was developed in these sirtuins and it was found that sirtuin activation actually prolongs longer life in yeast and then in mice.

In a study conducted in 2003, it was discovered that resveratrol found in red grape skin and red wine increases yeasts' lifespan. Studies have shown where resveratrol protects against the dangerous effects of increased fat, diets rich in sugar, high-calorie, increases fitness and also promotes healthy aging by putting age related diseases at bay first in mice and then in humans. As such, red wine became the first sirtfood, providing explanation of its benefits and why people who drink red wine seem to gain less weight.

These proteins are activated in the body through mild forms of stress, such as exercise and calorie restriction. Recent discoveries show that sirtuin activators are actually found in fruits and vegetables and carry out the same function as those in the body. Sirtfoods, as dubbed by authors and nutritionists Aidan Goggins and Glen are highly enriched with these sirtuin activators. When you bask in these main ingredients, the proteins encoded for by the SIRT1 gene, labelled as the "skinny gene" by Goggins and Matten is stimulated. It is safe to say that, if your diet comprises mainly of sirtfoods, you'll lose fat and also improve your health.

It is said that SIRT1 and sirtuin proteins are instrumental in aging and a longer life span, which might be identified with calorie restriction's protective effects. The case behind the Sirtfood Diet is that certain foods can actuate these pathways without the restriction and subsequently activate the body's ability to burn fat, speed up weight loss, and help fight off illnesses. The science on the sirtuin proteins is still fairly new. Research suggests that polyphenol-antioxidant resveratrol, an element in red wine, is linked to the weight management benefits of the sirtfoods.

You're probably wondering, why are there no supplement forms of sirtuin? In actuality, the mechanisms by which sirtuins operate are still not fully understood. It's believed that the body may not absorb the sirtuins in supplement forms as well as it does in its natural form.

Chapter 3
The Sirtfood Diet Plan

Phase One

The first phase of the Sirtfood Diet is regarded as the hyper-success phase as you aim towards the goal of a slimmer and leaner body. It lasts for one week and restricts the amount of calories consumed. For days one through three, a maximum of 1000 calories is allowed, where you consume three sirtfood green juices and one meal rich in sirtfood. The juices that are included are green tea, lemon juice, kale, rocket, parsley, celery, and green apples. Meals can include capers and parsley, chicken and kale curry, escalope with sage and prawn stir-fry with buckwheat noodles. On days four through seven, you should drink two sirtfood green juices and eat two sirtfood-rich meals, which should bring your calorie intake to a total of about 1500 per day.

The Sirtfood Diet is very big on green juice and is especially important in the first phase. It is composed of powerful sirtfood ingredients which contain a number of strong natural compounds such as apigenin, kaempferol, luetolin, quercetin and EGCG which work in unison to activate sirtuin genes and further promote fat loss. Nevertheless, you can also intake other fluids along with the recommended servings of green juice. These however, should be drinks that are noncaloric, such as water, coffee (black), or herbal tea. Coffee consumption however, should not entail any big changes as caffeine withdrawal symptoms can result in you feeling awful while increasing the amounts can make you to hyper.

It is within this phase, that you will obtain the full benefits of this clinically proven approach for losing seven pounds in just seven days. This phase also boasts muscle gain, so it is best not to weigh on a daily basis or get spun out on numbers. Because of muscle gain, you will see a change in the numbers when weighing but you will also see sustained waistline shrinkage. It is also recommended that you focus on your well-being, energy levels and your skin. Checks on your metabolic health, heart health are also encouraged to see if there are any differences in your blood glucose levels, blood pressure and blood fats. The sirtfood diet is not just weight reduction but also about taking a step in bettering your cells and resisting disease, for better lifelong health. The goal is to work the diet into your lifestyle and your day to day living for a more lengthened success.

For achieving the best outcome, we recommend:

1. Getting a good juicer: Juicing is very important to the sirtfood diet.
2. Prepare: Planning in advance gets you more results. Be sure to familiarise yourself with the different ingredients and recipes, and of course stock up on what you need.
3. Save Time: If you are one of those persons who tend to have a busy schedule, you can opt for preparing meals the night before, while juices can be done in bulk and refrigerated for as long as three days.
4. Eat Early: Eating earlier is better.
5. Space out Juices: Consume juices at least an hour before or even two hours after a meal to increase absorption.
6. Eat until Satisfied: Rather than forcing yourself to eat all the food, eat until you are satisfied. Sirtfoods do have quite an impact on appetite, where some persons before even finishing their meal they feel full.

7. Enjoy the Journey: Although you have an ultimate goal, focus on the journey. It is about the celebration of food and the health benefits that it poses all while enjoying it.

Seven Day Guide for Phase 1

Day 1

- Three sirtfood green juices
- One main meal (whether vegan or standard)

Standard:

- Asian shrimp stir-fry with buckwheat noodles
- ½ to ¾ ounce of dark chocolate (85% cocoa solids)

Vegan:

- Miso and sesame glazed tofu with ginger and chilli stir-fried greens with
- ½ to ¾ ounce of dark chocolate (85% cocoa solids)

Day 2

- Three sirtfood green juices

- One main meal

Standard:

- Turkey escalope with sage, capers and parsley and spiced cauliflower
- ½ to ¾ ounce of dark chocolate (85% cocoa solids)

Vegan:

- Kale and red onion dal with buckwheat with
- ½ to ¾ ounce of dark chocolate (85% cocoa solids)

Day 3

- Three sitfood green juices
- One main meal

Standard:

- Aromatic chicken breast with kale and red onions and a tomato and chilli salsa
- ½ to ¾ ounce of dark chocolate (85% cocoa solids)

Vegan:

- Harissa baked tofu with cauliflower
- ½ to ¾ ounce of dark chocolate (85% cocoa solids)

Day 4

- Two sirtfood green juices
- Two main meals

Standard:

- Sirt muesli
- Pan fried salmon fillet with caramelized endive, arugula and celery leaf salad.

Vegan:

- Sirt muesli
- Tuscan bean stew

Day 5

- Two sirtfood green juices
- Two main meals

Standard:

- Strawberry buckwheat tabbouleh
- Miso-marinated baked cod with stir-fried greens and sesame

Vegan:

- Strawberry buckwheat tabbouleh
- Soba (buckwheat noodles) in a miso broth with tofu, celery and kale.

Day 6

- Two sirtfood green juices
- Two main meals

Standard:

- Sirt super salad
- Char-grilled beef with a red wine jus, onion rings, garlic, kale and herb-roasted potatoes.

Vegan:

- Lentil sirt super salad
- Kidney bean mole with baked potato

Day 7

- Two sirtfood green juices
- Two main meals

Standard:

- Sirtfood omelette
- Baked chicken breast with walnut and parsley pesto and red onion salad

Vegan:

- Waldorf salad
- Roasted eggplant wedges with walnut and parsley pesto and tomato salad

Phase 2

The second phase, which is described as the maintenance phase, lasts for 14 days. This stage is designed for steady weight loss, and not just the maintenance of your current weight. During those two weeks, you are required to have three balanced sirtfood-rich meals and one sirtfood green juice daily. To be successful in phase two, your diet should be filled with sirtfoods.

There are still no set rules as to when these should be consumed. Flexibility is encouraged but it is suggested that you have your green juice in the morning, at least thirty minutes before breakfast, or even midmorning and do try to consume the evening meal before 7 pm.

The goal during phase two of the diet is to focus on sensible portions, well balance meal and packing your diet with sirtfoods to continue to reap the benefits they provide. Similarly to phase 1, it is important to listen to your body as your appetite guides you. Following these instructions and prepping meals according to such you will find that you'll be full before even finishing your meal. These sirtfoods when combined in your diet will naturally regulate your appetite as such the next fourteen days won't be spent feeling hungry.

In this phase, there is a continuation of a daily intake of green juice and similarly to phase one, you can consume other fluids as well. These fluids include plain water, homemade flavoured water, coffee, green tea and of course a glass of wine every now and then. Of course, the red wine should be within moderation, for example, one glass of red wine with a meal on two to three days per week.

Bringing back the three meals

Phase 1 consisted of the consumption of one or two meals per day and was adaptable in terms of when you ate meals. In going back to a more standard regime, and the practice of eating three meals a day, it is recommended that breakfast be one of those meals. Breakfast, helps us to start a new day, and ups our energy and focus levels. Many people tend to skip breakfast with the notion that they are too busy to prepare anything or we generally just don't have the time. The Sirtfood Diet plan however, has quite a few easy to whip up breakfast recipes. From the Sirtfood smoothie that can be consumed while you're on the go to the quick and easy scrambled eggs or tofu for vegans. Taking a few extra minutes in your morning routine will certainly prove beneficial to both your weight and health in the long term.

Sirtfoods really aim to energize us and an early morning intake of such will definitely get your day going. The green juice especially which can be had at least thirty minutes before breakfast in the mornings can result in you being less likely to feel hungry for a couple of hours; though this might have this effect, try your best not to opt out of breakfast.

Sirtfood Bites

Snacking is actually not as bad as it is sometimes made out to be. The Sirtfood Diet plan has a carefully put together menu which maintains a diet that will ensure a balanced three sirtfood rich meals a day. But there might be occasions where you find yourself wanting to have a snack as such the Sirtfood diet also comes with its own sirtfood bites. These of course are rich in sirtuin-activating nutrients and are also quite scrumptious. They are of course guilt-free and are made out of sirtfoods such as dates, walnuts, turmeric, extra virgin olive oil and cocoa. On the days that you find yourself needing these tasty little treats, it is recommended that you consume one or maximum two per day.

"Sirtifying" Meals

Sirtifying meals can be quite easy. It involves swapping out your non-Sirt rich foods fot ones rich in sirtuin activating nutrients, for example, kale, celery and strawberries.

As it relates to meat, it is recommended that you lessen your intake to two times a week. Additionally, it is advised that you either marinate the meat in Sirt rich foods such as olive oil, red onions and capers or serve alongside them. You can also cook your meat with food high in sirt, these include garlic, red onions, or even a cup of green tea will do.

To fully take advantage of the Sirtfood Diet, your meals should always be high in protein. Leucine a dietary protein stimulates Sirt1 which increases the burning of fat and improves blood glucose levels. It is also responsible for stimulating the build of cells within our bodies. Especially in muscle, which causes our mitochondria to work harder as it demands a lot of energy? A need for sirtuin activation is then developed as these will aid in the efficiency of the mitochondria so as to get them to burn more fat as fuel.

By combining proteins with Sirtfoods, there is a synergy where sirtuin activation is increased and more muscle growth takes place along with fat burn and overall better health. Leucine is found chiefly in animal protein; fish, seafood, eggs, dairy, red meat, and poultry. It is advised that you consume poultry instead of red meat. Studies have shown that the cancerous properties of meat are diminished when cooked with Sirtfoods, for example by adding an oil and or herb and keeping your consumption of meat as low as 1.5 pounds per week. While milk is restricted to a 1 liter per day, eggs and poultry however, can be eaten freely during the Sirtfood diet plan.

Oily fish are great to combine with your Sirtfood. They are high in omega 3 fatty acids, and also have some protein. Recent research suggests that the wide range of benefits of omega 3 fats may actually come intensifying how our sirtuin genes work. The best sources are herring, sardines, salmon, trout, mackerel, and tuna. You can supplement DHA for oily fish which has a high content of algae approximately 300mcg to be exact.

Chapter 4
What happens after finishing the Sirtfood Diet?

By now, you would have successfully completed both phases one and two of the diet and in doing so you've experienced a seven pounds weight loss and possibly some muscle gain. Additionally, you've further improved your body composition and maintained that weight loss all throughout the maintenance phase. Becoming leaner, toner and healthier.

The Sirtfood diet is not a one off diet but is instead a way of life. After completing the three weeks, there is no real set plan, but it is encouraged that you continue eating a diet rich in sirtfoods and drinking a green juice daily. It is all about tweaking one's lifestyle to include as many sirtfoods in your diet as possible which ultimately leads to you feeling healthier and more energetic in the long term. Although getting sweaty isn't the main focus of this diet plan, you are encouraged to exercise, with activities ranging from 30 minutes for five days per week.

Several sirtfood cookbooks can be found online as well as different recipes on the sirtfood website. One such recipe that can be found on the website is that of a combo of kale, parsley other leafy greens, celery, lemon juice, carrot, green apple, ginger, and matcha. Other ingredients recommended for use in your green juice are buckwheat and lovage. It is also urged that a juicer be used instead of a blender to enhance taste.

The Sirtfood Diet in Context

Written records of the benefits of sirtfoods date back to about 2200 years ago, in the book of Daniel in the Bible. To keep the young men healthy and fit, so they could successfully be a part of the King's service, were given a prescribed set of foods. However, it was questioned by Daniel, a plant-based diet was adopted and this showed better results. Such benefits included, increased muscle mass, with these plants being rich in sirtfood nutrients. Records show that the common plants consumed in those times, were actually similar to the Mediterranean diet which was rich in sirtfoods.

It is safe to say that back then, people were more concerned about curbing hunger than they were about weight. However things changed with the ancient Greeks, to have a beautiful mind, you had to have a body to match. There is a notable difference between then and now in relation to the idea of beauty. Women weren't seen as on the same level as men, physically, mentally or even emotionally as such, only men would boasts muscles and a toned figure.

When the Renaissance period came about, corsets became a big deal for women. The age of the corsets, is one to note as corsets were used to hide weight gain by the lacing corsets tighter and in those times, there was immense pressure to be thin and to remain that way. Many of these women would get sores from how tightly the corsets were laced and would eventually die when the sores got infected.

During the Renaissance period, the first diet book was published. Written by Luigi Cornaro, "The Art of Living Long",who at the age of 40 was overweight, portrayed his strategy of weight reduction. This included him restricting himself to fourteen ounces of wine per day with twelve ounces of food. Cornaro's diet comprised of bread, egg yolks, meat and soup with wine and in being somewhat successful he losing some pounds, he decided to write a book about it, which is quite popular. Cornaro actually lived a longer life dying at maybe 98 or 102 years of age. Is it safe to say that Cornaro might have piloted the sirtfood diet?

Giacomo Castelvestro, published the book "The Fruits Herbs and Vegetables of Italy" in 1614. This book encourages the eating of not just vegetables but also herbs and fruits. Could Castelvestro be a foreather of the sirtfood diet? There are several of his recipes that are included in the sirtfood diet recipe book.

How is the Sirtfood Diet Different from other Diets?

What makes the sirtfood diet plan different? Is it just another fad or diet craze? There are a wide range of diet plans out there to choose from. But at the end of the day, the decision is up to you and choosing what works best for you. Dieting is usually hard, and there are many conflicting information out there regarding diets. If you are going to follow a new diet plan, what you can do and evaluation based on other diet programs.

The Sirtfood diet is very much different from various other diet plans that are out there. Why? Because with the Sirtfood diet, you won't see a pronounce weight loss. You will instead notice a stable reduction in fat that will offer promising long term health benefits. However, before you embark on any dietary journey, be sure to talk with a health practitioner.

Sirtfoods are great for dietary plans, and overall provide considerable benefits in terms of weight and health. This is in relation to diet plans that include fasting, low fat, paleo and gluten free diets which have been enormously growing practices. The Sirtfood diet plan boasts similar to or even more favourable outcomes than severe sporadic fasting.

The 20 sirtfoods within the Sirtfood diet plan are all used in their natural state and as such more promising when it comes on to having a nutritious diet plan. The plan is different from others as it allows for the body to burn fat at a faster pace and doesn't make a big deal of calorie restriction. With that said, you can journey on a weight loss plan that doesn't ask you to starve yourself nor engage in rigorous exercise because it provides you with the advantages of both without having to do either.

Whilst exercise and fasting does activate the sirtuins, your exercise regimen does not have to be anything severe, and to be honest, there are many who no matter how healthy they want to be, cannot engage in rigorous exercise. The Sirtfood diet only includes a very mild-fasting, for fasting for long periods of time or even long term can be quite dangerous as it restricts the intake of nutrients. In consuming sirtfoods, you can better your health while building muscle without any harm.

Sirtfoods and other Foods

Incorporating several other foods in your sirtfood diet has been proven to be advantageous. When mixed together, they can provide a higher boost in health. With foods that are rich in polyphenol, helping to prevent or reduce inflammatory diseases such as cardiovascular diseases, imagine combining other nutrition packed foods to your die. Here are a few types of the foods that may create optimum effect.

Green tea with lemon: the ingredients in green tea contain flavonoids antioxidants such as catechins, and epigallocatechin gallate (EGCG) which provide numerous potential health benefits, including heart disease and cancer preventions, as well as weight loss benefits. Adding lemon improves the health benefits of the tea by bringing out the antioxidants, making them more available for absorption. Lemon juice can significantly up the amount of catechins that your body extracts from the green tea by approximately up to six times.

Tomato and Extra virgin olive oil: These superfoods protect, energize and satiate but when combined together, they amplify each other's benefits. Tomatoes contain the antioxidant lycopene which gives it its beautiful red color, and also prevents heart diseases and prevent certain types of cancer for example, prostate, breast, lung and bladder cancer. The body however, has a hard time absorbing lycopene if the tomato is raw. So to get the nutrients it contains, it is best to cook the tomato, combining it with oil. The extra virgin olive oil is a great choice as it results in maximum absorption.

Turmeric and black pepper: also known as the golden spice, turmeric is a tall plant that grows in Asia and Central America. It has been used in traditional Indian cooking, for thousands of years, to treat many different health conditions. The most active ingredient in turmeric the polyphenol, curcumin has several advantages to health. It is a strong antioxidant and anti-inflammatory, antibacterial and antifungal properties. But its greatest downfall is the inability to absorb effectively in the body. Black pepper on the other hand contains piperine which has been shown to help relieve nausea and headaches, is beneficial in boosting the absorption of curcumin, making them the most ideal spice couple.

Looking Beyond the Twenty Sirtfoods

Evidently, the sirtfoods are quite advantageous. The top twenty sirtfoods are foods that are bulked with sirtuin-activating compounds, producing end results in the body such as increased burning of fat leading to weight loss and an overall healthier well-being. Nevertheless, there are multiple other plants that also produce some levels of these activating nutrients, you can of course include these as a part of your diet and reap the benefits.

Let's look at berries for instance, one of the top twenty sirtfoods are strawberries, known for its richness in the sirtuin-activating nutrient fisetin. If we examine the berries food group on a wider scale, we discover that they are highly beneficial in metabolic health and encouraging healthy aging. Berries such as blueberries, raspberries, and blackberries have rmearkable levels of sirtuin-activating compounds. Similarly with nuts, though they are high in calories, they help to prevent the risk of chronic diseases and also aid in weight loss removing a few inches from the waistline. Sirtuin-activating nutrients are also found in chestnuts, peanuts, pistachios and pecans.

Studies have shown a correlation between consuming whole-grain and the positive effects of reduced inflammation, heart disease, cancer and diabetes. Whole-grains other than buckwheat do contain sirtuin-activating nutrients but when these whole-grains are processed into refined versions, they lose their sirtuin-activating compounds and instead become harmful. Other wholegrains that have sirtfood properties are qunioa (gluten-free), cha seeds and goji berries. Popcorn, yes popcorn is also a great whole-grain sirtfood snack.

There are forty other foods that have been found to contain sirtfood properties, you can make these a part of your dieting, nourishing it with even more sirtuin-activating nutrients which will help in managing weight loss and improve well-being. These forty foods include:

Vegetables

- Asparagus
- Artichokes
- Green Beans
- Pak Choi/ Bok Choy
- Broccoli
- Shallots
- Frisee
- Watercress
- White Onions
- Yellow Endive

Fruits

- Black currants
- Black plums
- Red Grapes

- Raspberries
- Goji Berries
- Apples
- Cranberries
- Kumquats
- Blackberries

Nuts and seeds

- Sunflower Seeds
- Chia Seeds
- Peanuts
- Chestnuts
- Pecan Nuts
- Pistachio Seeds

Grains and Pseudo-Grains

- Quinoa
- Popcorn
- Whole-wheat Flour

Herbs and Spices

- Cinnamon
- Dil (fresh and dried)

- Dried Oregano
- Thyme (fresh and dried)
- Ginger
- Peppermint (fresh and dried)
- Chives
- Dried Sage

Beans

- White Beans
- Fava Beans

Beverages

- White Tea
- Black Tea

The Power of Proteins

It has been discovered that a diet high in protein is beneficial as it reduces muscle mass loss, manages metabolism and promotes satisfaction. When combined with Sirtfoods, it produces even more favourable benefits.

Protein is vital in the Sirtfood diet. It is comprised of amino acids and the amino acid leucine works together with Sirtfoods, to further improve their effects. How is this achieved? It does so by fundamentally altering our cellular environment and thus the sirtuin-activating nutrients function much more effectively. Poultry, red meat, seafood, fish, eggs and dairy are primary sources of leucine.

Animal-Based Protein

Animal based products have been dubbed as a contributing factor to many diseases within the Western regions, specifically that of cancer. The animal products that are complete sources of protein include fish, dairy products, such as milk, cheese and whey, eggs, red meat from cows, poultry from chickens and turkeys, and meat from horses and hares. The animal-based proteins are made up of saturated fats and increased levels of cholesterol. Dairy products stimulate mTOR in the body (mammalian target of rapamycin) which is linked to aging and the growth of age related disorders such as cancer, neurodegenerative illnesses, type II diabetes and obesity.

If Sirtfoods are added to a diet consisting of dairy products, then the undesirable effects that mTOR have on our cells are hindered thus diminishing the danger. A diet rich in Sirtfood and containing dairy products in moderation poses no known risks and even offer multiple useful nutrients when combined. Dairy is a beneficial source of protein and a great source of vitamins such as calcium, phosphorous and iodine. But it is recommended that adults consume up to three helpings, no more than 1 litre of dairy a day.

There is considerable evidence pointing to increased health risks of consuming red and processed meat, especially hot dogs, ham, and pepperoni; these health risks include colorectal cancer, breast cancer and even prostate cancer. We're not saying that you should cut it out of your diet completely, it should however, be consumed in small portions. Research has shown that combining them with Sirtfoods actually cancels the risk of cancer. You can combine these within your Sirtfood diet by marinating with herbs, extra virgin olive oil, and spices. Beef especially can be cooked with onions or you can go further and add a cup of green tea with the meal. It is recommended that adults consume maximum three servings of red meat a week.

The Power of Three

The omega-3 fatty acids dates back to observational studies conducted in the late 1970's within the Greenland Inuits. The Eskimo population had low rates of coronary heart disease and this was credited to their traditional diet consisting of marine animals and fish; all rich in omega-3 fatty acids called EPA and DHA. Other studies show where the Alaskan and Japanese cultures which have similar diets rich in fish consumption have similarly low rates of death caused by coronary heart disease.

Known best for their nutritional benefits, omega-3 fatty acids provide great results when combined with Sirtfoods. A group of sirtuin genes that are correlated with longevity are enhanced by these fatty acids. They have various health benefits, the most prominently known heart health benefits coupled with the reduction of inflammation as well as the fat levels in the blood. With omega-3s, the likelihood of blood clotting is reduced and the electrical rhythm of the heart kept at a stable pace, as well as decreasing blood pressure levels.

Omega-3s are found in fish especially the oily varieties. To observe the great benefits of omega-3s, eat two servings of oily fish each week. Omega-3s are also found in plant foods such as nuts, seeds, and green leafy vegetables, however, in the form of alpha-linolenic acid, which needs to be converted to EPA or DHA in the body. But the conversion is not a sufficient enough and as such only provides limited amount of the omega3-s.

The most valuable omega-3 fish sources are herring, sardines, salmon, trout, and mackerel, in that order. For vegetarians and vegans, while plant sources should still be a part of your diet, it is however recommended that a supplement of DHA-enriched microalgae be consumed.

The Effect of Physical Activity

There are multiple health benefits linked to being active and these are reduced risk of cardiovascular disease, stroke, hypertension, type 2 diabetes, osteoporosis, obesity, and cancer. Physical activity or exercise also improves one's mood, sleep cycle their overall well-being. Exercise actually complements a diet rich in Sirtfoods. There are many advantages of turning on our "skinny genes", but that doesn't mean we should not engage in physical activities.

Exercise maximizes the stimulation of sirtuin-activating nutrients in the body and provides a wide array of benefits. As such it is encouraged that you follow the guideline of the two hours and 30 minutes where you engage in moderate physical activity each week. Or you can also engage in 75 minutes of aerobic activity per week. You can also combine both.

Moderate-intensity physical activities include dancing or brisk walking for at least 2.5 miles per hour. You can partake in other sporting activities as well but ultimately, these activities increase your heart rate and are beneficial as they improve cardiorespiratory fitness.

Another important aspect is reducing sitting time. The more hours spent sitting each day the more you are prone to metabolic issues. Too much sitting can negatively affect your health and longevity. You can go biking, do some gardening or if you are someone with pets for example dogs, you can take him for a walk or throw a ball around in a game of fetch.

No matter the form of physical activity that you partake in, it counts, especially when performed on a daily basis and at a moderate intensity. Physical activity gets your sirtuin genes activated and thus further increasing the benefits of the Sirtfood diet plan. Exercise plus eating a diet rich in Sirtfoods provides you with the maximum level of sirtuin activation.

Chapter 5
Pros and Cons of a Sirtfood Diet

Pros

- The twenty sirtfoods listed in the sirtfood diet are known for being advantageous to health.
- With the research done on sirtuin, it is shown where heightened levels of sirtuin proteins lead to prolong life in organisms such as yeast, worms and mice.
- You can see positive results within a short period of time
- It is an inclusive diet, meaning, it allows the combining of foods rich in sirtuin-activating nutrients and other foods rich in various other nutrients.
- Vegan recipes are also available
- Recipes are adaptable
- You are able to retain and gain muscle while losing weight

Cons

- Depending on where you're located, some foods might be harder to source, for example matcha green tea, lovage and buckwheat
- A juicer is needed if you don't already own one
- There are not many scientific studies readily available on the sirtfood diet

Arguments against the Sirtfood diet include:

- Evidence supports the notion that calorie restriction can lead to loss of muscle.
- Calorie restriction might make it difficult for some people to keep up the diet
- The diet is restrictive

Is The Sirtfood Diet For You?

There is no weight loss or dieting plan for everyone. But if you are to take into consideration your lifestyle, preferences and goals, you'll likely find a plan that suits your needs.

The Sirtfood diet plan allows you to drop weight, maintain and or gain muscle, and feel healthier. The first couple of weeks can be challenging and it is utmost important that you evaluate which foods are best to eat and which of the recipes are more suited for you.

You're probably wondering how much does this cost? If there are supplements, do you have to visit a weight loss clinic, or even attend support meetings? There will always be some amount of expense or challenge or risks even, when it comes on to a dieting program.

Before deciding on a diet plan it is also talk to your doctor. Research has shown where what works for one person may not work for another.

The best weight loss plan is the one you can keep up. With that in mind, if you which to follow the sirtfood diet plan or any plan for that matter, consider the following:

- Your personal needs: diet's you've already tried
- Your personal preferences

- You're budget
- Age and sex
- Sleep patterns
- Environmental factors
- Psychological Factors
- You're activity level
- You're job
- Cooking facilities
- Family needs
- Cultural beliefs
- Spiritual beliefs

Whether you decide to partake in this diet plan or another, consult other studies and ensure it is in keeping with what you would like to achieve. Monitor your progress, your wins and losses and weigh them against each other. If you find yourself having more losses than wins, then the diet may not be for you.

Frequently asked Questions

Are Sirtfoods suited for kids?

The Sirtfood diet can be just an effective weight loss diet program for kids, though it was not specifically designed for them. With that in mind, there are quite a number of the recipes that were created with families in mind. The green juice, however isn't recommended as it contains a high concentration of fat burning sirtfoods.

Should I exercise throughout Phase 1?

Exercising regularly is one of the best practices that can benefit your health.

Partaking in repeated moderate exercise can improve fat loss and the wellness benefits of phase 1 of the plan. While exercise is encouraged, it is advised that during this period the degree of exercise not be too heavy or extreme exercise puts stress on the body. Instead do only what you are comfortable with and listen to your body.

Is the Sirtfood Diet science-based?

Though research has been done as it relates to the benefits of sirtuins, there is little to no research in regards to the Sirtfood dietary plan. If you are concerned about the safety of the sirtfoood diet plan, many if not all of the sirtfood that were listed are known to have nutritious benefits, as proven by scientific research.

Can I still follow the diet even though I am already slim?

To anyone who is underweight, the Sirtfood diet is not recommended. The best method of finding out if you are underweight is by calculating your body mass index (BMI). Once you are aware of your height and your weight, then you can successfully ascertain your BMI by making used of the many BMI calculators that are readily available on the internet. A BMI between 18.5 and 20 is not extremely low but be cautious as in following the Sirtfood diet it is highly possible that your BMI may drop below 18.5. Being underweight can have adverse effects on various aspects of health, such as a lowered immune system and the heightened risk osteoporosis which is the weakening of the body's bones.

You can however, still integrate a rich amount of sirtfoods into a balanced diet so as to benefit from all the health advantages they provide. You can most certainly partake in the Sirtfood diet, if you are slim and have a BMI of 20 to 25. Quite a number of the persons who participated in the pilot study had healthy BMIs; however, they still had impressive amounts of weight loss, became toner and reported notable enhanced energy levels, vitality and image.

Is the Sirtfood Diet for obese persons?

A small number of persons who participated in the Sirtfood diet pilot study were obese and actually had even better outcomes than the participants who had a healthier weight. Obesity poses quite a number of health risks such as chronic heart problems so why not embark on a diet journey where you can reap the benefits of protection from such helath problems.

Should I stop eating Sirtfoods once I've reached my target weight?

The further restriction of calorie intakes is not recommended during this time but it is advised that one's diet remain consistent in Sirtfoods. Sirtfoods are a way of life, helping you to manage your weight and health so you look and feel good.

Can pregnant women follow the diet?

If pregnant, trying to get pregnant or breastfeeding, undertaking this diet journey is not encouraged as the

Sirtfood diet is a powerful in weight loss. One can however, still eat plenty of Sirtfoods, as they are remarkably healthy foods that can be incorporated as part of a balanced diet during pregnancy. Because of its alcohol content, steering clear of red wine is advised. Similarly it is encouraged that if you do include Sirtfoods in your diet during pregnancy, then you should check those foods that contain caffeine such as coffee, green tea and cocoa. It is advised that no more than 200 milligrams of caffeine be consumed during pregnancy. Also only four cups of green tea should be consumed daily and the matcha green tea should definitely be avoided.

Once Phase 2 is completed Do I Stop Drinking the Morning Sirtfood Green Juice?

The morning green juice is a great way to start the day as such it is encouraged that this be consumed long term. The Sirtfood diet green juice contains ingredients that boast a high level of sirtuin-activating nutrients that promote the burning of fat and improves well-being. Nevertheless, you don't have to continue consuming the morning juice but it is recommended to reap long term benefits.

Can persons who take medication follow the diet?

Though the Sirtfood diet is appropriate for most people, its powerful outcomes on burning fat and health can actually negatively impact certain disease processes and actions of prescribed medication, similarly to how some medications are not fitting for during the fasting. In conducting the Sirtfood diet trial, each person was assessed in terms of whether or not they were suitable to take part in the diet, with special attention on those persons who were on medication. In cases of persons suffering from crucial health problems, persons on prescribed medications, it is recommended that a discussion be had with their doctor before embarking on the Sirtfood diet. It is always important to check with your doctor first before beginning any diet plan especially if you have any medical conditions. Your doctor can help to guide you along your weight loss journey and make sure that this diet plan is right for you.

Chapter 6
Meal Plans and Recipes

A Sirtfood Diet Meal Plan

With the principles in mind, here's a menu that can be used during the maintenance phase (phase 2).

For breakfast, you can have:

- Omelette (kale)
- Muesli (mixture of oats and other cereals, dried fruit and nuts)
- Strawberries and yoghurt
- Fruit smoothie made from soy milk and rolled oats

For lunch and dinner, you can have:

- A rocket salad made up of tuna, cucumber (dressed in olive oil), and tomatoes
- A spicy tofu-stir fry inclusive of bird's eye chilli, packed with veggies
- Fish (grilled) and buckwheat salad

- Stir fried chicken and soba
- Tofu burgers and salad (wholegrain bread)
- Kale salad with red onions and edamame beans (dressed in olive oil)
- Spicy curry chicken with a serving of wholegrain brown rice

Snacks included are:

- Dark Chocolate
- Coffee
- Fresh fruit (strawberries)
- Celery
- Walnuts
- Dark chocolate

Recipes

Green Juice

Serves 1

Ingredients:

- 2 large handfuls (about 2 ½ ounces or 75g) kale

- A large handful (1 ounce or 30g) rocket/arugula
- A very small handful (about ¼ ounce or 5g) parsley
- 2 to 3 large celery sticks (5 ½ ounces or 150g), including the leaves
- ½ medium green apple
- ½ to 1 inch (1 to 2.5cm) piece of fresh ginger
- Juice of ½ lemon
- ½ teaspoon matcha powder

HOW TO MAKE:

- It is best to use a juicer, as recommended to have the desired effect.
- Mix the kale, arugula and parsley together, and then juice them. The goal is to have about 2 fluid ounces or close to ¼ cup (50ml) of juice from the greens.
- Now juice the celery, apple and ginger.
- Squeeze the lemon by hand into green juice. By this time you should have about 1 cup (250ml) of juice or more.
- Then add a small amount of the green juice into a glass and stir in the matcha.

- Add the remainder of the green juice into the glass and stir once more.

Sirtfood Bites

Ingredients:

- 120g walnuts
- 30g dark chocolate (85% cocoa) broken into pieces
- Pitted medjool dates (250g)
- 1 tablespoon cocoa
- 1 tablespoon ground turmeric
- 1 tablespoon extra-virgin olive oil
- 1 teaspoon scraped seeds of a vanilla pod
- 1-2 tablespoon water

HOW TO MAKE:

- Place chocolates and walnuts into a food processor and process until it turns into a fine powder.
- Apart from the water, add all other ingredients and blend until the mixture forms into a ball.
- Mould the mixture into bit-size balls using your hands and put on the refrigerator in an

airtight container for approximately one hour before consuming.

Strawberry Buckwheat Tabbouleh

Serves 1

Ingredients:

- 1/3 cup (50g) buckwheat
- 1 tbsp ground turmeric
- ½ cup (80g) avocado
- 3/8 cup (65g) tomato
- 1/8 cup (20g) red onions
- 1/8 (25g) Medjool dates, pitted
- 1 tbsp capers
- ¾ cup (30g) parsley
- 2/3 cup (100g) strawberries, hulled
- 1 tbsp extra virgin olive oil
- Juice of ½ lemon
- 1 ounce (30g) arugula

HOW TO MAKE:

- Cook buckwheat with turmeric according to the package instructions.

- Drain and put aside to cool.
- Finely chop avocado, tomato, red onion, dates, capers, and parsley and mix together with the cooled buckwheat.
- Then slice the strawberries and gently mix into the salad with the oil and lemon juice.
- Serve on a bed of arugula.

Aromatic chicken breast with red onions, kale and a tomato and chilli salsa

1 Serving

Ingredients:

- ¼ pound (120g) skinless, boneless chicken breast
- 2 tsp ground turmeric
- Juice of ¼ lemon
- 1 tbsp extra virgin olive oil
- ¾ cup (50g) kale, chopped
- 1/8 cup (20g) red onion, sliced
- 1 tsp chopped fresh ginger
- 1/3 cup (50g) buckwheat

For the Salsa

- 130g tomato (about 1)
- 1 bird's eye chilli, finely chopped
- 1 tbsp capers, finely chopped
- 2 tbsp (5g) parsley, finely chopped
- ¼ of lemon juice

HOW TO MAKE:

When making the salsa the eye from the tomato should be removed and chopped finely, retaining as much liquid as possible. You then mix the capers, lemon juice, parsley and chilli together.

- Heat oven to 220°C.
- Chicken breast should be marinated in 1 teaspoon of the turmeric, a little olive oil and the lemon juice. Leave for approximately 5-10 minutes.
- Then heat an ovenproof frying, when hot add marinated chicken and cook for 1 minute on each side, until pale golden.
- Transfer to the oven and leave for 8-10 minutes to cook right through. Remove from

oven and cover with foil and leave to rest for about 5 minutes before serving.
- In the meantime, put kale to cook in the steamer for approximately for 5 minutes.
- Fry red onions and the ginger in a little oil, until they are soft, then add the kale and fry for one more minute.
- Cook buckwheat according to packet instructions with the remaining teaspoon of turmeric.
- Serve alongside the chicken, vegetables and salsa.

Stir Fried Asian with Buckwheat Noodles

1 Serving

Ingredients:

- 1/3 pounds (150g) raw jumbo shrimp (shelled), deveined
- 2 tablespoon tamari
- 2 teaspoon extra virgin olive oil
- 3 ounces (75g) buckwheat noodles
- 2 garlic cloves, finely chopped
- 1 Thai chilli, finely chopped

- 1 teaspoon finely chopped fresh ginger
- 1/8 cup (20g) red onions, sliced
- ½ cup (45g) celery with leaves (trimmed and sliced)
- ½ cup (75g) green beans, chopped
- ¾ cup (50g) kale, roughly chopped
- ½ cup (100ml) chicken stock

HOW TO MAKE:

- Over high heat, heat a frying pan and then cook shrimp in 1 teaspoon of oil and 1 teaspoon of tamari for a total of 2 to 3 minutes.
- Transfer shrimp to a plate.
- Clean pan with a paper towel for use once more.
- Cook the noodles for 5 to 8 minutes in boiling water as directed on packaging. Drain and then set aside.
- In the meantime, fry the garlic, chilli, red onions, celery (leaves not included), kale and green beans in the remainder of tamari and oil over medium to high heat for 2 to 3 minutes.

- Then add stock and bring to boil, shimmer for a minute or two, until vegetables are cooked but are still crunchy.
- Add shrimp, noodles and celery leaves to the pan, bring back to a boil, then remove and serve.

Sirt Super Salad

Serves 1

Ingredients:

- 1 ¾ ounces (50g) arugula
- 1 ¾ ounces (50g) endive leaves
- 3 ½ ounces (100g) smoked salmon slices
- ½ cup (80g) avocado, peeled, stoned and sliced
- ½ cup (50g) celery including the leaves, sliced
- 1/8 cup (20g) red onions, sliced
- 1/8 cup (15g) walnuts, chopped
- 1 tablespoon capers
- 1 large Medjool date, pitted and chopped
- 1 tablespoon extra-virgin olive oil
- Juice of ¼ lemon
- ¼ cup (10g) parsley, chopped

HOW TO MAKE:

- Place salad leaves on a plate or within a large bowl.
- Combine and mix all the remaining ingredients together and serve on top of the leaves.

Miso-Marinated Baked Cod with Stir-Fried Greens and Sesame

Serves 1

Ingredients:

- 3 ½ teaspoon (20g) miso
- 1 tablespoon mirin
- 1 tablespoon extra-virgin olive oil
- 1 x 7 ounce (200g) skinless cod fillet
- 1/8 cup (20g) red onions, sliced
- 3/8 cup (40g) celery, sliced
- 2 garlic cloves, finely chopped
- 1 Thai chilli, finely chopped
- 1 teaspoon finely chopped fresh ginger
- 3/8 cup (60g) green beans
- ¾ cup (50g) kale, roughly chopped

- 1 teaspoon sesame seeds
- 2 tablespoon tamari
- ¼ cup (40g) buckwheat
- 1 teaspoon ground turmeric

HOW TO MAKE:

- Mix miso, mirin and 1 teaspoon of the oil together. Then rub all over the cod and leave to marinate for 30 minutes.
- Heat the oven at 220 °C. Bake the cod for 10 minutes.
- In the meantime, bring a large frying pan or wok to with the remainder of the oil. Add the onion and let it stir-fry for a few minutes, then add the kale, celery, garlic, chilli, green beans and ginger.
- Toss until the kale is tender and cooked right through.
- Cook the buckwheat according to packet instructions together with the turmeric.
- Add the sesame seeds, tamari and parsley to the stir-fry and serve with the buckwheat and fish.

Breakfast Recipes

Sirtfood mushroom scrambled eggs

Ingredients

- 1 teaspoon ground garlic
- 1 teaspoon mild curry powder
- 20g lettuce, sliced
- 1 teaspoon extra virgin olive oil
- ½ bird's eye peeled, thinly chopped
- A couple of mushrooms, finely chopped
- 5g parsley, finely chopped

HOW TO MAKE:

- Mix curry and garlic powder then add a little water until you've achieved a light glue.
- Steam lettuce for two to 3 minutes.
- In a skillet, heat oil over a moderate heat and fry the chili and mushrooms two to three 3 minutes until they've begun to soften and brown.
- Add the eggs and spice paste and cook over a medium heat then add the carrot and proceed to cook over a moderate heat for a further

minute. In the end, put in the parsley, mix well serve.

Blue Hawaii smoothie

Ingredients

- Two tablespoon rings or approximately 4-5 balls
- ½ cup frozen tomatoes
- Two tablespoon ground flaxseed
- ⅛ cup tender coconut (unsweetened, organic)
- A few walnuts
- ½ cup fat-free yogurt
- 5-6 ice cubes
- Splash of water

HOW TO MAKE:

- Put all of the ingredients together and combine until smooth.

Turkey breakfast sausages

Ingredients

- 1 lb extra lean ground turkey

- 1 tablespoon extra-virgin olive oil, and a little more to coat pan
- 1 tablespoon fennel seeds
- 2 tsp smoked paprika
- 1 teaspoon red pepper flakes
- 1 teaspoon peppermint
- 1 tsp chicken seasoning
- A couple of shredded cheddar cheese
- A couple of chives, finely chopped
- A few shakes garlic and onion powder
- Two spins of pepper and salt

HOW TO MAKE:

- Preheat oven to 180 °C.
- Utilize a little EVOO to dirt grease a miniature muffin pan.
- Combine all ingredients and blend thoroughly.
- Fill each pit on top of the pan and then cook for approximately 15-20 minutes. Each toaster differs

Banana pecan muffins

Ingredients

- 3 tablespoon butter softened
- 4 ripe bananas
- 1 tablespoon honey
- ⅛ cup OJ
- 1 teaspoon cinnamon
- 2 cups all-purpose pasta flour
- 2 capsules
- A couple of pecans, sliced
- 1 tablespoon vanilla

HOW TO MAKE:

- Preheat the oven to 180°C
- The bottom and sides of the muffin tin should be lightly greased and then dusted with flour.
- Dust the surfaces of the tin gently with flour then tap to eradicate any excess.
- Peel and insert the batter to a mixing bowl and with a fork, mash the carrots so that you've got a combination of chunky and smooth, then put aside.

- Insert the orange juice, melted butter, eggs, vanilla and spices and stir to combine.
- Roughly chop the pecans onto a chopping board, and then fold throughout the mix.
- Spoon of the batter ¾ full and bake in the oven for approximately 40 minutes, or until golden and cooked through.

Banana and blueberry muffins

Ingredients

- 4 large ripe bananas, peeled and mashed
- ¾ cup of sugar
- 1 egg, lightly crushed
- ½ cup of butter, melted (and a little extra to dust the interiors of this muffin tin)
- 2 cups of blueberries (if they are frozen, do not defrost them, simply pop them into the batter suspended as is)
- 1 teaspoon baking powder
- 1 teaspoon baking soda
- ½ teaspoon salt
- 1 cup of coconut bread
- ½ cup of flour (or 1-1; two cup bread)

- ½ cup applesauce
- A dash of cinnamon

HOW TO MAKE:

- Add mashed banana to a large mixing bowl.
- Add sugar & egg and mix well.
- Add peanut butter and strawberries.
- Sift all the dry ingredients together then add the dry ingredients into the wet mix and mix together lightly.
- Set into 12 greased muffin cups
- Bake for 20-30min in 180c or 350 f.

Morning meal sausage gravy

Ingredients

- 1 lb sausage
- 2 cups 2 percent milk (complete whole milk is great also)
- ¼ cup entire whole wheat bread flour
- Salt and a lot of pepper to flavour

HOW TO MAKE:

- Cook sausage from skillet.
- Add flour and blend cook for about a minute.
- Add two cups of milk.
- Whisk whilst gravy thickens and bubbles.
- Add pepper and salt and keep to taste until perfect.
- Let stand a minute or so to
- To dish, scrape it over several snacks or desired foods.

Easy egg-white muffins

Ingredients

- English muffin
- Egg-whites - 6 tbsp or two large egg whites
- Turkey bacon or bacon sausage
- Sharp cheddar cheese or gouda
- Green organic berry
- Optional- lettuce, and hot sauce, hummus, flaxseeds, etc...

HOW TO MAKE:

- Get a microwavable safe container, then spray entirely to stop the egg from adhering, then pour egg whites into the dish.
- Lay turkey bacon or bacon sausage paper towel and then cook.
- Subsequently, toast your muffin, if preferred.
- Then put the egg dish in the microwave for 30 minutes. Afterward, with a spoon or fork, immediately flip egg within the dish and cook for another 30 minutes.
- Whilst the dish remains hot, sprinkle some cheese while preparing sausage.
- The secret is to get a paste of some kind between each coating to put the sandwich together, i.e. - a very small bit of hummus or even cheese.

Sweet potato hash

Ingredients

- Inch 1 sweet-potato
- ½ red pepper, diced
- 3 green onions, peppermint

- Leftover turkey, then sliced into bits (optional)
- 1 tablespoon of butter
- Carrot powder - a few shakes
- Pepper - only a small dab
- Pepper and salt to flavour
- Sprinkle of shredded cheddar cheese (optional)

HOW TO MAKE:

- Poke a sweet potato and microwave for 5 minutes.
- Remove from microwave, peel skin off and chop.
- In a skillet, on medium-high heat, place peppers and butter and sauté for a few minutes.
- Insert potato bits and keep sautéing.
- Whilst you sauté, add sweeteners, leafy vegetables, and green onions.
- Insert a dab of cheddar and revel in the taste!

Asparagus, mushroom artichoke strata

Ingredients

- 1 Inch loaf of sourdough bread
- 4 challah rolls
- 8 eggs
- 2 cups of milk
- 1 teaspoon salt
- ¼ teaspoon black pepper
- 1 cup fontina cheese, cut into little chunks
- ½ cup shredded parmesan cheese
- 1 tablespoon butter
- 1 teaspoon dried mustard
- ½ can of artichoke hearts, sliced
- 1 bunch green onions, grated
- 1 bunch asparagus, cut into 1-inch bits
- 1 10oz package of baby Bella (cremini) mushrooms, chopped

HOW TO MAKE:

- Clean mushrooms and slice and trim asparagus cutting it into 1-inch pieces. Reserve Place in a bowl and scatter ½ teaspoon salt mixture.

- Drain and dice ½ or medium artichoke hearts.
- Melt butter in a pan over moderate heat, also sauté the asparagus and mushrooms before the mushrooms start to brown. Do this for, about 10 minutes.
- Blend the artichoke core pieces into a bowl with all a mushroom/asparagus mix. Set aside.
- Cut or split a tiny sourdough loaf into 1-inch bits.
- Grease a 9x13 inch baking dish and generate a base coating for bread in the dish. Spread ½ cup of fontina cheese on bread, as a coating, and disperse half an apple mixture and green onions on the cheese.
- Lay-down a different layer of these vegetables and bread using a ½ cup of fontina cheese.
- Whisk together eggs, salt, milk, dry mustard, and pepper into a bowl, and then pour the egg mixture on the vegetables and bread.
- Cover the dish, and then simmer for 3 hours.
- Preheat oven to 375 degrees.
- Remove the casserole from the fridge and let stand for half an hour.

- Spread all the parmesan cheese at a coating within the layers.
- Bake in preheated oven then insert a knife near the border (must come out clean, 40 to 45 minutes. Let cool for approximately 5 to 10 minutes then cut into squares.

Egg white veggie wontons w/fontina topped w/ crispy prosciutto

Ingredients

- 1 cup egg whites
- Butter
- Fontina cheese
- Mixed shredded cheddar cheese
- Broccoli I utilized wheat, chopped bits
- Tomatoes – diced
- Salt and pepper
- Prosciutto - two pieces
- Won ton

HOW TO MAKE:

- Remove won ton wrappers out of the freezer.
- Preheat oven to 350.

- Spray miniature cupcake tin with cooking spray.
- After wrappers begin to defrost, peel them off carefully, one at a time and press in cupcake tin lightly.
- Slice the wrappers having adding a little bit of peanut butter (optional).
- Set a chunk of cheese on the bottom.
- Add desired lettuce and vegetables
- Pour egg whites and all toppings.
- Sprinkle each with some of those shredded cheddar cheese.
- Cook for approximately 15 minutes, but watch after 10 minutes - whenever they poof up - assess them by poking the middle with a fork.
- While eggs are cooking, spray a sheet of foil with cooking spray and then put 2 two pieces of prosciutto onto it and then cook at exactly the exact same period time as the egg whites. After 8 minutes, take them from the heat and let sit. Once it cools, it becomes crispy. Chop and add on top of eggs.

Crunchy and chewy granola

Ingredients

- Two ¼ cup old-style yogurt
- 1 Inch tablespoon flax seeds
- ¼ teaspoon kosher salt
- ½ teaspoon cinnamon
- ¼ ground ginger
- ½ cup honey
- Two tablespoon packaged splendid brown-sugar
- ¾ cup ounces raw peppers
- ½ cup sliced peppers
- ½ cup golden raisins
- ½ cup dried cranberries
- 1 tablespoon vanilla sugar (to make put a used vanilla bean in a full bowl of sugar and allow to simmer in freezer.

HOW TO MAKE:

- Preheat oven to 300.
- Line baking sheet with parchment paper.
- Mix 9 components together.

- Insert 1 cup hot tap water, and then use your hands to mix together and spread into a thin coating over a baking sheet.
- Bake for 60 minutes, stirring 2-3 minutes, before turning black gold brown.
- Remove from the oven and let cool.
- Stir in dried fruit.
- Dust with sugar.

Blueberry pancakes

Ingredients

- 2 eggs
- 1 cup milk
- 1 tablespoon vegetable oil
- 1.5 tsp butter melted, (and an additional piece of peanut butter to the pan)
- Inch ¼ cup all-purpose flour 3 tsp baking powder
- 3 teaspoon sugar
- ½ teaspoon salt
- 2 cups frozen blueberries

HOW TO MAKE:

- Put a non-stick griddle or a skillet over moderate heat.
- Independent eggs yolks and whites, moving whites to some medium mixing bowl.
- Whisk functions well with milk, butter, and oil.
- Gradually fold dry ingredients to liquid with a wooden spoon.
- In yet another bowl, sift together dry skin.
- Working with an electric beater, whip egg whites until frothy.
- Pour egg whites into the batter (small lumps of egg white are fine).
- When skillet is hot, brush the skillet with melted butter.
- Pour ¼ cup batter onto the skillet for each pancake, leaving space.
- Top each pancake using 5- 6 blueberries.
- When bubbles form inside the batter, flip the pancake.
- Keep on cooking until golden brown, for about two minutes.
- Eat instantly.

Power balls

Ingredients

- 1 cup old fashion ginger, dried
- ¼ cup quinoa cooked using 3/4 cup orange juice
- ¼ cup shredded unsweetened coconut
- 1/3 cup dried cranberry/raisin blend
- 1/3 cup dark chocolate chips
- ¼ cup slivered almonds
- 1 tablespoon reduced-fat peanut butter

HOW TO MAKE:

- Cook quinoa in orange juice. Bring to boil and simmer for approximately 1-2 minutes. Let cool.
- Combine chilled quinoa, and the remaining ingredients into a bowl.
- With wet hands combine ingredients and roll in golden ball sized chunks.
- Set at a Tupperware and set in the refrigerator for two hours until firm.

Cinnamon crescent rolls

Ingredients

- 2 refrigerated crescent rolls
- 1 stick butter, softened
- ½ cup brown or white sugar
- 1 tablespoon cinnamon
- Glaze
- ½ cup powdered sugar
- 1 teaspoon vanilla
- 2 tablespoon milk

HOW TO MAKE:

- Heat oven to 350°f.
- In a small bowl mix sugar, butter, and cinnamon; beat until smooth.
- Separate dough into rectangles.
- Add on each rectangle about two tablespoon cinnamon butter mix.
- Roll-up starting at the broadest side, as you'll ordinarily do to crescent rolls. Firmly press ends to seal.

- Put each cinnamon filled crescent roll on a parchment line-up baking sheet. *be sure that you line the cookie sheet or you might have a huge mess after *
- Bake for approximately 10 to 15 minutes or until golden brown in colour.
- In a small bowl, combine all glaze ingredients, adding enough milk for desired drizzling and consistency. Drizzle over hot rolls.

Fresh fruit pizza

Ingredients

- 4 crescent rolls (rolled-out and poked with a fork)
- Two spoonsful of moderate cream-cheese
- Inch 1 teaspoon of sugar
- 1 teaspoon vanilla extract
- Handful berries - chopped (you can easily utilize lemon, blueberries or beer)
- Sliced almonds

HOW TO MAKE:

- Place crescent rolls in a non-stick pan and then poke a few times with a fork. Cook at 375 for approximately 14 minutes. Let cool.
- In a bowl combine cream, vanilla extract & and sugar. Stir with a spoon.
- Spread onto crescent rolls, then add almonds and fruit.

LUNCH RECIPES

Sticky chicken watermelon noodle salad

Ingredients

- 2 pieces of skinny rice noodles
- ½ tablespoon sesame oil
- 2 cups watermelon
- Head of bib lettuce
- Half of a lot of scallions
- Half of a lot of fresh cilantro
- 2 skinless, boneless chicken breasts
- ½ tablespoon Chinese five-spice
- 1 tablespoon extra-virgin olive oil
- 2 tablespoon sweet skillet

- 1 tablespoon sesame seeds
- A couple of cashews – smashed
- Dressing
- 1 tablespoon low-salt soy sauce
- 1 teaspoon sesame oil
- 1 tablespoon peanut butter
- ½ a refreshing red chili
- ½ a couple of chives
- ½ a couple of cilantros
- 1 Inch limes – juiced
- 1 small spoonful of garlic

HOW TO MAKE:

- In a bowl, completely submerge the noodles in boiling drinking water.
- On a big sheet of parchment paper, sprinkle the chicken with pepper, salt and spice.
- Twist over the paper, and flatten the chicken using a rolling pin.
- Place into the large skillet with 1 tablespoon of olive oil, turning 3 or 4 minutes, until well charred and cooked through.

- Drain noodles and toss with 1 tablespoon of sesame oil onto a sizable serving dish.
- Place 50% of the noodles into the skillet, stirring frequently until crispy and nice.
- Remove the watermelon skin, then slice the flesh into inconsistent balls and then move to plate.
- Wash the lettuces and cut into small wedges and also half of a whole lot of leafy greens and scatter on the dish.
- Place another ½ the cilantro pack, the soy sauce, coriander, chives, peanut butter, and a dab of water, 1 teaspoon of sesame oil and the lime juice in a bowl, then mix till smooth.
- Set the chicken back to heat and garnish with all the sweet sauce and then toss with the sesame seeds.
- Pour the dressing on the salad, toss gently with fresh clean fingers until well coated, then add crispy noodles and then smashed cashews.
- Mix chicken pieces and add them to the salad.

Fruity curry chicken salad

Ingredients

- 4 skinless, boneless chicken pliers - cooked and diced
- 1 teaspoon celery, diced
- 4 green onions, sliced
- 1 inch peeled apples, cored and diced
- 1/3 cup golden raisins
- 1/3 cup seedless green grapes, halved
- ½ cup sliced toasted pecans
- ⅛ teaspoon ground black pepper
- ½ teaspoon curry powder
- ¾ cup light mayonnaise

HOWTO MAKE:

- In a big bowl combine the chicken, onion, celery, apple, pecans, pepper, curry powder, and carrot. Mix altogether.

Zuppa Toscana

Ingredients

- 1 lb majority medium ground Italian sausage
- 1 ¼ teaspoon crushed red pepper flakes
- 4 pieces bacon, cut into 1/2½ inch bits
- 1 big onion, diced
- 1 tablespoon minced garlic
- 5 (13.75 oz) can chicken broth
- 6 celery, thinly chopped
- 1 cup thick cream
- ¼ bunch fresh spinach, tough stems removed

HOW TO MAKE:

- Cook that the Italian sausage and red pepper flakes in a toaster pot on medium-high heat until crumbly, browned, with no longer pink, 10 to 15minutes. Drain and put aside.
- Cook bacon until crispy over medium heat, about 10 minutes. Drain, leaving a couple of tablespoons of drippings. Together with all the bacon at the bottom of the toaster. Stir in the

garlic and onions and then cook until onions are tender and translucent, about five minutes.
- Pour the chicken broth into the toaster pot with the onion and bacon mix; contribute to a boil on high temperature. Add the berries, and boil until fork-tender, about 20 minutes. Lower heat to medium and stir in the cream and also the cooked sausage. Mix the lettuce to the soup before serving.

Turmeric chicken & kale salad with honey-lime dressing

Ingredients

For your poultry

- 1 teaspoon ghee or 1 tablespoon coconut oil
- ½ medium brown onion, diced
- 250 to 300 grams / 9 oz. Chicken mince or chicken thighs
- 1 large garlic clove, finely chopped
- 1 teaspoon turmeric powder
- 1 teaspoon lime zest (optional)
- juice of ½ lime
- ½ teaspoon salt

For your salad

- 6 broccoli 2 or two cups of broccoli florets
- 2 tablespoon pumpkin seeds
- 3 big kale leaves, stalks removed and sliced
- ½ avocado, chopped (optional)
- bunch of coriander leaves, chopped
- couple of fresh parsley leaves, chopped

For your dressing

- 3 tablespoon lime juice
- 1 small garlic clove (finely diced or grated)
- 1 tablespoon extra-virgin coconut oil
- 1 teaspoon raw honey
- ½ teaspoon whole grain or dijon mustard
- ½ teaspoon sea salt and salt

HOW TO MAKE:

- Heat coconut oil in a small skillet pan above medium-high heat. Bring the onion and then sauté on medium heat for 45 minutes, until golden. Insert the chicken blossom and garlic and

simmer for 2-3 minutes on medium-high-heat.
- Add the garlic, lime zest, lime juice, and salt and soda and cook, stirring often, to get a further 3-4 minutes. Place the cooked mince aside.
- As the chicken is cooking, add a little spoonful of water. Insert the broccoli and cook 2 minutes. Rinse under warm water and then cut into 3-4 pieces each.
- Insert the pumpkin seeds into the skillet and chicken placed chicken in over medium heat for two minutes, stirring often to avoid burning. Season with a little salt.
- Put chopped spinach in a salad bowl and then pour over the dressing. With hands, massage and toss the carrot with the dressing. This will dampen the lettuce.
- Finally, toss the cooked chicken, broccoli, fresh herbs, pumpkin seeds, and avocado pieces.

Buckwheat noodles with chicken kale & miso dressing

Ingredients

For the noodles

- 2 to 3 handfuls of kale leaves
- 150 g / 5 ounce buckwheat noodles (100 percent buckwheat, no wheat)
- 3 to 4 shiitake mushrooms, chopped
- 1 tsp coconut oil or ghee
- 1 brown onion, finely diced
- 1 medium free-range chicken, chopped or diced
- 1 red chili, thinly chopped (seeds out based on how hot you want it)
- 2 large garlic cloves, finely chopped
- 2 to 3 tablespoon tamari sauce (fermented soy sauce)

For miso dressing

- 1 inch or 2½ tablespoon fresh organic miso
- 1 tablespoon tamari sauce

- 1 tablespoon peppermint oil
- 1 tablespoon lime or lemon juice
- 1 teaspoon sesame oil (optional)

HOW TO MAKE:

- Bring a medium saucepan of water. Add the kale and cook 1 minute, until slightly wilted. Remove and put aside but keep the water and put it back to boil. Insert the soba noodles and cook according to the package directions (usually about five minutes). Rinse under warm water and place aside.
- Meanwhile, pan fry the shiitake mushrooms and just a very little ghee or coconut oil (about a tsp) for 23 minutes, until lightly browned on each side. Sprinkle with sea salt and then place aside.
- In the same skillet, warm olive oil ghee over medium-high heat. Sauté onion and simmer for 2 3 minutes and add the chicken bits. Cook five minutes over medium heat; stirring a few

times, you can put in the garlic, tamari sauce and just a tiny dab of water. Cook for a further 2-3 minutes, stirring often until chicken is cooked through.

- Lastly, add the carrot and soba noodles
- Mix the miso dressing and scatter on the noodles before eating; in, this manner, you can retain dozens of enzymes that are beneficial

Baked salmon salad with creamy mint dressing

Ingredients

- 1 salmon shrimp (130g)
- 40g mixed salad leaves
- 40g young spinach leaves
- 2 radishes, trimmed and thinly chopped
- 5cm slice (50g) cucumber, cut into balls
- 2 spring onions, trimmed and chopped

- 1 small number (10g) parsley, roughly sliced

To the dressing

- 1 teaspoon low-fat mayonnaise
- 1 tablespoon organic yogurt
- 1 tablespoon rice vinegar
- 2 mint leaves, finely chopped
- Salt and freshly ground black pepper

HOW TO MAKE:

- Pre heat the oven to 200°c (180°c fan/gas 6).
- Two set the salmon fillet onto a baking dish and bake for 16--18 minutes until cooked. Remove from the oven and place aside. The salmon is every bit as fine cold or hot in the salad.
- In a small bowl, combine together the mayonnaise, yogurt, rice vinegar, coriander leaves, and salt and salt together and leave to stand for at least 5 minutes to permit the

- A arrange the salad leaves onto the serving plate and top with the radishes, cucumber, spring onions, and parsley. Flake the carrot on the salad and drizzle the dressing.

Choc processor granola

Ingredients:

- 200g jumbo oats
- 50g pecans
- Chopped
- 3 tablespoon olive oil
- 20g butter
- 1 tablespoon dark brown sugar
- 2 tablespoon rice malt syrup
- Darkened chocolate chips

HOW TO MAKE:

- Preheat the oven to 160°C.
- Line a large baking pan with a silicone sheet or parchment paper.
- In a large bowl, add oats and pecan and mix together.

- In a small skillet, gently warm the coconut oil, butter, brown sugar, and rice malt before the butter melts and the sugar and butter have simmered. Don't let it boil. Pour the syrup on the ginger and stir thoroughly before the oats are wholly covered.
- Distribute the granola within the skillet, dispersing straight into the corners. Leave clumps of mix with spacing. Bake in the oven for about 20 minutes until edges are a tinge of golden brown. Take from the oven and put to cool.
- When cooled, divide some larger lumps onto the plate together with your palms and mix in the chocolate chips. Twist or put the granola in an airtight jar or tub.

Fragrant Asian hotpot-Sirtfood recipes

Ingredients:

- 1 teaspoon tomato purée

- 1 star of anise, crushed (or even 1/4 tsp ground anise)
- Small amount (10g) of parsley, stalks finely chopped
- Small amount (1og) coriander, stalks finely sliced
- Juice of all ½ lime
- 500ml chicken stock, fresh or left using inch block
- ½ carrot, peeled and cut into match sticks
- 50g broccoli, cut into small florets
- 50g beansprouts
- 100g raw tiger prawns
- 100g firm carrot, sliced
- 50g rice noodles, cooked as per packet directions
- 50g cooked chestnuts, drained
- 20g sushi ginger, sliced
- 1 tablespoon high miso glue

HOW TO MAKE:

- Put the chicken stock, tomato purée, star anise, parsley stalks, coriander stalks, and carrot juice in a large pan and simmer for approximately 10 minutes.
- Add the lettuce, prawns, tofu, noodles, and water chestnuts and simmer gently until the prawns are cooked through. Remove from heat and stir in the skillet along with miso paste.

Lamb, butternut squash and date tagine

Ingredients

- 2 teaspoon coconut oil
- 1 red onion, chopped
- 2cm ginger, grated
- 3 garlic cloves, crushed or grated
- 1 teaspoon chili flakes (or to taste)
- Cumin seeds (2 teaspoon)
- 1 stick of cinnamon
- 2 teaspoons turmeric (ground)

- lamb neck fillet (800g) cut in chunks of 2cm
- ½ teaspoon salt
- 100g Medjool dates, pitted and sliced
- 400g tin chopped berries, and half of a can of plain water
- 500g butternut squash, chopped into 1cm cubes
- 400g tin chickpeas, drained
- 2 teaspoon fresh coriander (and extra for garnish)
- Buckwheat, couscous, flatbread or rice to serve

HOW TO MAKE:

- Preheat oven to 140C.
- Drizzle roughly tablespoon of coconut oil into a large ovenproof saucepan or cast-iron casserole dish. Add the chopped onion and cook on a gentle heat, with the lid for around five minutes, just to soften the onions..

- Add the grated ginger and garlic, chili, cumin, and cinnamon. Stir well and cook 1 minute with the lid off. Add a dash of water when it becomes too dry.
- Next, the lamb balls. Stir to coat the beef meat with the spices and onions then add the salt, chopped meats, dates and berries, and roughly half of a cup of plain water (100-200ml).
- Bring the tagine into to boil and with the lid and on your skillet for about 1 hour and fifteen minutes.
- Ten minutes prior to the end of this cooking time, add the chopped butternut squash and drained chickpeas. Stir together, and put the lid back on and put back in the oven to the last half an hour of cooking.
- When can be removed from the oven, stir fry throughout the chopped coriander. Add buckwheat, couscous, flat pieces of bread or basmati rice.

Prawn arrabbiata

Ingredients

- 125-150 g beef or cooked prawns (ideally king prawns)
- 65-gram buckwheat pasta
- 1 tablespoon extra- virgin coconut oil
- 40 g red onion, finely chopped
- 1 garlic clove, finely chopped
- 30-gram celery, thinly sliced
- 1 bird's eye chili, finely chopped
- 1 teaspoon dried mixed veggies
- 1 tablespoon extra-virgin coconut oil
- 2 tablespoons white wine (optional)
- 400 gram tinned chopped berries
- 1 tablespoon chopped parsley

HOW TO MAKE:

- Fry the garlic, onion, celery and peppermint blossoms in the oil over medium-low heat for 1 to 2 minutes. Turn heat to medium, and cook the wine for 1 second. Add the berries and let the sauce simmer over medium-low heat for 20 minutes to half an hour, until it's a great rich texture. In the event, you're feeling that the sauce is becoming too thick, simply put in little water.

- As the sauce is cooking, set a bowl or pot of water to the boil and then cook the pasta as per the package directions. Once cooked, drain, then toss with the olive oil.
- If you're utilizing raw prawns put them into your sauce and cook for a further 3 to 4 minutes, until they've turned opaque and pink, then add the parsley. If you're using cooked prawns add them to the skillet, then bring the sauce to boil.
- Add the cooked pasta into the sauce, then mix thoroughly but lightly and serve.

Turmeric baked salmon

Ingredients

- 125-150 grams of skinned salmon
- 1 tablespoon extra-virgin coconut oil
- 1 teaspoon ground turmeric
- ¼ juice of a lemon
- 1 teaspoon extra virgin coconut oil
- 40g red onion, finely chopped
- 60g tinned green peas
- 1 garlic clove, finely chopped
- 1 cm fresh ginger, finely chopped
- 1 bird's eye chili, finely chopped
- 150 gram celery, cut into 2cm lengths
- 1 teaspoon darkened curry powder
- 130 gram tomato, cut into 8 wedges
- 100 ml vegetable or pasta stock
- 1 tablespoon chopped parsley

HOW TO MAKE:

- Heat the oven to 200°C.
- Heat a skillet over a moderate medium --low heat, then add the olive oil then

the garlic, onion, ginger, celery, and peppermint. Fry lightly for two to three minutes until softened but not coloured, add curry powder and cook for a another minute.

- Put in berries, afterward your lentils and stock and simmer for 10 seconds. You might choose to increase or reduce the cooking time according to how crunchy you'd like your own sausage.
- In the meantime, mix the olive oil, garlic and lemon juice and then rub the salmon. Set on the baking dish and cook 8--10 seconds.
- Stir in the celery and serve with the salmon.

Coronation steak salad

Ingredients

- 75 g natural yogurt
- Juice of ¼ of a lemon
- 1 teaspoon coriander, sliced

- 1 teaspoon ground turmeric
- ½ teaspoon darkened curry powder
- 100g cooked chicken, cut to bite-sized pieces
- 6 walnut halves, finely chopped
- 1 Medjool date, finely chopped
- 20g crimson pumpkin, diced
- 1 bird's eye chilies
- 40 gram rocket, to serve

HOW TO MAKE:

- Mix the lemon, carrot juice, spices, and coriander together in a bowl. Add all the remainder of ingredients and serve on a bed of rocket.

Baked potatoes with spicy chickpea stew

Ingredients

- 4 to 6 celery sticks, pricked all-over
- 2 teaspoon coconut oil
- 2 red onions, finely chopped
- 4 cloves garlic, crushed or grated

- 2 cm ginger, grated
- 2 ½ teaspoons chili flakes
- 2 tablespoons cumin seeds
- 2 teaspoon turmeric
- Splash of water
- 2 (400g) tins chopped tomatoes
- 2 tablespoons unsweetened cocoa powder
- 2 (400g) tins chickpeas with the chickpea water
- 2 yellow peppers, chopped into bite-size pieces
- 2 tablespoons parsley and extra for garnish
- Salt and pepper to taste (optional)

HOW TO MAKE:

- Preheat the oven to 200°C.
- When the oven is still hot enough set your lemon potatoes in the oven and cook for 1 hour or so.
- Remove the potatoes from the oven, place the coconut oil and sliced red

onion into a large wide saucepan and cook lightly, with the lid for five minutes until the onions are tender but not brown.

- Remove the lid and then add the ginger, garlic, cumin, and simmer. Cook for a further minute on very low heat, then add the garlic and a tiny bit of water and then cook for another moment, just take care never to allow the pan to get too warm.
- Next, add the berries, cocoa powder (or even cacao), chickpeas (including the chickpea water) and salt. Bring to boil, and then simmer on a very low heat for 4 to 5 seconds before the sauce is thick and unctuous (but do not allow it to burn up). The stew has to be prepared at exactly the exact same time as the legumes.
- Finally, stir in the two tablespoon of parsley, plus a few pepper and salt if you desire, and also serve the stew in addition to the chopped sausage, possibly with a very simple salad.

Kale and red onion dhal with buckwheat

Ingredients

- 1 tablespoon coconut oil
- 1 small red onion, chopped
- 3 garlic cloves, crushed or grated
- 2 cm lemon, grated
- 1 birds eye chilli, deseeded and finely chopped
- 2 teaspoon turmeric
- 2 teaspoons gram masala
- 160g red lentils
- 400ml coconut milk
- 200ml water
- 100g kale (or lettuce)
- 160g buckwheat (or brown rice)

HOW TO MAKE:

- Put the coconut oil in a large, deep saucepan and then add the chopped onion. Cook on very low heat, with the lid for five minutes until softened.

- Add garlic, ginger, and chili; cook for one minute.
- Add the garlic, gram masala and a dash of water and then cook for 1 minute.
- Add the reddish peas, coconut milk, and also 200ml water (try so only by half filling the coconut milk with water and stirring it in the saucepan).
- Mix everything together thoroughly and then cook for 20 minutes over light heat with the lid on. Stir occasionally and add just a little bit more water in case the dhal starts to stick.
- After 20 seconds, add the carrot, stir thoroughly and then replace the lid, then cook for a further five minutes (1 to 2 minutes if you are using spinach)
- Around 1 to 5 minutes when the curry is ready, set the buckwheat at a medium saucepan and then put in lots of warm water. Bring back the water to the boil and then cook for 10 minutes (or only a little longer in case

you would rather your buckwheat softer. Drain the buckwheat using at a sieve and serve with the dhal.

Char-grilled steak having a dark red wine jus, onion rings, garlic kale, and herb-roasted potatoes

Ingredients:

- 100g potatoes, peeled and cut into 2cm
- 1 tablespoon extra-virgin coconut oil
- 5g parsley, finely chopped
- 50g red onion, chopped into circles
- 50g lettuce, chopped
- 1 garlic clove, finely chopped
- 120 to 150g (3.5cm) thick beef noodle or 2cm-thick sirloin beef
- 40ml red wine
- 150ml beef stock
- 1 teaspoon tomato purée
- 1 teaspoon cornflour- dissolve in 1 tablespoon of water

HOW TO MAKE:

- Heat the oven to 220°C.
- Put the sausage in a saucepan of boiling water, then return to boil and then cook 4 minutes, then empty. Put in a skillet with 1 tablespoon of the oil and then roast in the oven for 3 to 5 minutes. Stir the berries every 10 minutes to ensure even cooking. After cooking, remove from the oven, sprinkle with the chopped parsley and mix well.
- Fry the onion with 1 tsp of the oil over a medium heat for 5 minutes for 1 minute, until tender and well caramelized. Maintain heat. Steam the kale for two to three minutes. Stir the garlic lightly in ½ tsp of oil for 1 minute, until tender but not coloured. Let spinach simmer for another 1 to 2 minutes, until tender. Maintain heat.
- Heat an ovenproof skillet on high heat until smoking. Put the beef in ½ a tsp of the oil and then fry in the skillet

over a medium-high temperature in accordance with how you would like your beef done. If you prefer your beef medium it'd be wise to sear the beef and also transfer into a toaster place in 220°c/petrol 7 and then finish the cooking in whichever way you like.

- Set meat aside to rest.
- Add wine to the skillet to bring up any meat up residue. Simmer to decrease the wine for half an hour until syrupy along with a flavour that is concentrated
- Add the stock and tomato purée into the beef pan and bring to the boil, to thicken the sauce, adding it only a little at a time until you've got your preferred consistency. Stir in just about any of those juices and serve with the roasted lettuce, celery, onion rings, and red berry sauce.

Kale and black-currant smoothie

Ingredients

- 2 teaspoon honey
- 1 cup freshly made green tea
- 10 baby spinach leaves, stalks removed
- 1 ripe banana
- 40g blackcurrants washed, and stalks removed
- 6 ice cubes

HOW TO MAKE:

- Stir the honey into the green tea before dissolved.
- Blend each of the ingredients together in a blender until smooth. Drink instantly.

DINNER RECIPES

Bang-bang chicken noodle stir-fry recipe

Ingredients

- 1 tablespoon sunflower oil
- 750g package chicken thighs, boned
- 250g frozen chopped mixed peppers
- 1 inch courgette, peeled into ribbons, seeded and chopped
- 1 chicken stock cube
- 250g pack medium egg yolks
- 4 garlic cloves, finely chopped
- ½ teaspoon crushed chilies
- 4 tablespoons reduced-salt soy sauce
- 2 teaspoon caster sugar
- 1 lime, zested, ½ juiced, ½ sliced into wedges to serve

HOW TO MAKE:

- On medium-low heat, add oil to skillet. Fry the chicken skin for 10 mins or until crispy. Flip and simmer for 10 mins, or until cooked. Add to a plate and use a foil wrapper to loosely cover.

- Reheat the wok over a high temperature, add the peppers and sliced courgette; simmer for 5 mins. Meanwhile, bring a bowl of water to the boil, and then crumble in the stock block, adding the noodles. Simmer for 45 mins until cooked, and then drain.
- Add the garlic and crushed chilies into the wok; simmer for two mins. Mix sugar, soy, lime juice and zest in a bowl. Enhance the wok, boil for 2 minutes, you can add the courgette noodles and ribbons. Use tongs to toss and sauce.
- Cut the chicken into pieces. Divide the noodles into four bowls and top with the chicken. Serve with the lime wedges along with extra crushed chilies.

Cajun steak and veg rice jar

Ingredients

- 1 tablespoon vegetable oil
- 1 celery stick, finely chopped
- 3 large carrots, sliced into rounds
- 250g frozen chopped mixed peppers
- 4 chopped spring onions
- 500g 5 percent beef mince
- 2 teaspoon seasoning
- 1 teaspoon tomato purée
- 2 x 250g packs ready-cooked long-grain rice

HOW TO MAKE:

- Over medium heat, add a large shallow skillet and heat oil. Add the carrots, celery, peppers and snowy areas of the frozen peppers. Cook for 10 minutes before the vegetable is beginning to soften.

- Add the mince, season and cook for 10 minutes before mince is browned and start to really get crispy.
- Add the Cajun seasoning and tomato purée; stir fry to coat the mince. Place inside with the rice, combined with 4 tablespoons of plain water. Stir to completely combine until the rice is hot. Sprinkle on the rest of the spring onion before serving.

Pesto salmon pasta noodles recipe

Ingredients

- 350g penne
- 2 x 212g tins cherry salmon, drained
- 1 lemon, zested and juiced
- 190g jar green pesto
- 250g package cherry tomatoes halved
- 100g bunch spring onions, finely chopped
- 125g package reduced-fat mozzarella

HOW TO MAKE:

- Preheat the oven to 220°C. Boil the pasta for five minutes. Drain, reserving 100ml drinking of the pasta water.
- Meanwhile, in a 2 ltr ovenproof dish, mix the salmon, lemon zest and juice, then pesto, berries and half of the spring onions; season.
- Mix the pasta. Mix the remaining pesto using 1 tablespoon water and then drizzle on the pasta. Gently sprinkle with the mozzarella, top with the rest of the spring onions and bake for 25 minutes until golden.

Sri Lankan-style sweet potato curry

Ingredients

- ½ onion, roughly sliced
- 3 garlic cloves, roughly sliced
- 25g sliced ginger, chopped and peeled
- 15g fresh coriander stalks and leaves, sliced

- Two ½ tablespoon medium curry powder
- 60g package cashew nuts
- 1 tablespoon olive oil
- 500g Red Mere farms sweet potatoes, peeled and cut into 3cm balls
- 400ml tin isle sun coconut-milk
- ½ vegetable stock block, as much as 300ml
- 200g grower's harvest long-grain rice
- 300g frozen green beans
- 150g Red Mere farms lettuce
- 1 sun trail farms lemon, ½ juiced, ½ cut into wedges to serve

HOW TO MAKE IT:

- Set the onion, ginger, garlic, coriander stalks and tikka powder along with half of the cashew nuts in a food processor. Add 2 tablespoons water and blitz into a chunky paste.
- In a large skillet, warm the oil over medium heat. Add the paste and cook, stirring for 5 mins. Put in the sweet

- potatoes, stir, then pour in the coconut milk and stock. Bring to simmer and boil for 25 to 35 mins before the sweet potatoes are tender.
- Meanwhile, cook the rice, following packet directions. Toast the rest of the cashews in a dry skillet.
- Stir the beans into the curry and then simmer for two minutes. Add the lettuce in handfuls, allowing each to simmer before adding the following, lemon juice, to taste, & and the majority of the coriander leaves. Sprinkle on the remaining coriander and cashews. Serve with the rice and lemon wedges.

Chicken liver along with tomato ragu

Ingredients

- 2 tablespoon olive oil
- 1 onion, finely chopped
- 2 carrots, scrubbed and simmer
- 4 garlic cloves, finely chopped

- ¼ x 30g pack fresh ginger, stalks finely chopped, leaves ripped
- 380g package chicken livers, finely chopped
- 400g tin grower's harvest chopped berries
- 1 chicken stock cube, created around 300ml
- ½ teaspoon caster sugar
- 300g penne
- ¼ sun trail farms lemon, juiced

HOW TO MAKE:

- In a large skillet, heat 1 tablespoon oil over medium-low heat. Fry the onion and carrots for 10 minutes, stirring periodically. Stir in the ginger and garlic pops cloves and cook for more minutes. Transfer into a bowl and set aside.
- Turn the pan on high heat and then add the oil. Add the chicken livers and simmer for 5 mins until brown. Pour the onion mix into the pan and then

stir in the tomatoes, sugar, and stock. Season, bring to boil, and then simmer for 20 mins until reduced and thickened, and the liver is cooked through. Meanwhile, cook pasta to package guidelines.

- Taste the ragu and put in a second pinch of sugar or more seasoning, if needed. Put in a squeeze of lemon juice to taste and stir in two of the shredded basil leaves. Divide the pasta between four bowls, then spoon across the ragu and top with the rest of the basil.

Minted lamb with a couscous salad recipe

Ingredients

- 75g couscous
- ½ chicken stock block, composed to 125ml
- 30g pack refreshing flat-leaf parsley, sliced
- 3 mint sprigs, leaves picked and sliced
- 1 tablespoon olive oil

- 200g pack suspended bbq minted lamb leg beans, de-frosted
- 200g lettuce berries, sliced
- ¼ teaspoon, sliced
- 1 spring onion, sliced
- Pinch of ground cumin
- ½ lemon, zested and juiced
- 50g reduced-fat salad cheese

HOW TO MAKE:

- Add couscous to a heatproof bowl. Pour out contents then cover and put aside for at least 10 minutes, then using a fork and stir in the herbs.
- Rub a little oil on the lamb steaks and season in the meantime. Cook to package guidelines then stir.
- Mix cucumber, tomatoes and spring onion in the couscous with oil, the cumin, and lemon juice and zest. Crumble on the salad and serve with the lamb.

Jack fruit tortilla bowls recipe

Ingredients

- Two sweet corn cobettes
- 1 red chili, finely chopped
- Two teaspoons of olive oil
- 1 juiced lime
- Chopped fresh coriander (15g)
- packaged stained jack fruit in sauce (150g)
- 210g tin kidney beans, drained
- 125g roasted red peppers (in the jar), drained and chopped
- Two whitened tortilla packs
- ½ round lettuce, ripped

HOW TO MAKE:

- On a high temperature, heat a griddle pan. Griddle the cobettes for 10 to 12 minutes, turning until cooked and charred throughout. Remove from the pan. Use a sharp knife to carefully reduce the span of this corn, staying near to the heart, to clear away the kernels. Mix that the kernels with the eucalyptus oil, half of the carrot juice along with half an hour of the coriander.

- Heating the jack fruit and sauce in a saucepan with the legumes, peppers, lime, coriander and juice on medium-low heating for 3 to 4 minutes until heated through.
- Griddle the wraps for 10 to 20 seconds, each side to char. Tear into pieces and serve together with all the jack fruit, lettuce and sweet corn salsa.

Carrot, courgette and halloumi hamburgers recipe

Ingredients

- 1 big carrot, grated
- 1 large courgette, grated
- 225g halloumi, grated
- 2 spring onions, finely chopped
- 90g bread crumbs

- 1 tablespoon ground cumin
- 1 tablespoon ground coriander
- ½ teaspoon salt
- 2 tablespoon flour
- 4 brioche buns, halved
- 50g baby spinach leaves
- 1 big tomato, sliced
- 1 small red onion, chopped
- ½ pineapple, peeled into ribbons
- Tzatziki, to serve

HOW TO MAKE:

- Put the courgette tea towel and squeeze to eradicate any liquid. Place into a big bowl and then add the carrot, halloumi, onion, bread crumbs, cumin, coriander, eggs, salt, and flour. Stir well to mix.
- Put over half the mix in a food processor until the mixture starts to stick. Combine this into the mix.
- Divide the mix into four and then form into patties. Heat a grill or

griddle pan on medium heat. Cook the hamburgers for 45 mins, each side until golden and cooked through.

- Add the hamburger buns into the grill till lightly toasted. To assemble the burgers, put lettuce leaves on the base of each bun. Top with all the hamburgers, a piece of tomato, pineapple ribbon along with a spoonful of tzatziki.

Rita's 'rowdy' enchiladas recipe

Ingredients

- Two large chicken breasts (about 400g)
- 2 red peppers, thinly chopped
- 1 tablespoon olive oil
- ¾ teaspoon mild chili powder
- ½ teaspoon ground cumin
- ¾ teaspoon smoked paprika
- 80g grated mozzarella
- 8 plain tortilla wraps
- 5g ripe cheddar, grated

- 10g fresh coriander, roughly sliced

For the sauce

- 1 tablespoon olive oil
- ½ onion, finely chopped
- 2 teaspoon cloves, crushed
- 500g tomato pasta
- 1 tablespoon chipotle chili paste
- 400g tin black beans drained and rinsed
- ½ lime, juiced

HOW TO MAKE:

- Preheat the oven to 190°c. Set the chicken in a 20 x 30cm skillet with all the peppers olive oil, chili powder, cumin, and paprika. Mix to coat, then cover with foil. Roast for 25 to 30 mins before the chicken is cooked and tender until no pink meat remains. Take out the chicken from the dish and shred with two forks. Reserve in a bowl.

- Meanwhile, make the sauce. Heat the oil in a saucepan on a low heat and cook the garlic and onion for 10 mins. Stir in the pasta and chipotle chili glue; increase heat to medium, simmer and then cook for another 10 minutes, stirring from time to time. Use the beans and carrot juice to season.
- Mix one-third of this sauce plus half of the mozzarella with the broccoli and chicken.
- Spoon 4 tablespoons of this sauce in the same baking dish as before. Spoon a bit of the chicken mixture down the middle of each tortilla, roll up and then put in the dish. Repeat with the tortillas and filling, then placing them alongside so they do not shatter. Pour the remaining sauce on the top and then sprinkle the remainders of the cheddar and mozzarella. Bake in oven for approximately 20 to 25 mins until the cheese melts and starts to brown. Sprinkle with all the coriander to serve.

Freezing and defrosting recommendations

Cook as instructed and let it cool completely. Subsequently move to an airtight, freezer-safe container, seal and freeze up to 1 to 3 weeks. Ensure that the meatballs are underwater in the sauce so they can freeze better. To serve, defrost thoroughly in the refrigerator overnight before reheating. To serve, put in a bowl over medium heat, stirring occasionally until the dish is heated throughout.

Full-of-veg hash

Ingredients

- 2 red onions, finely chopped
- 300g carrots, peeled and diced
- Two courgettes, diced
- 2 garlic cloves, crushed
- 4 eggs
- 5g refreshing flat-leaf parsley, sliced
- 1 red chili, chopped (optional)
- ½ x 340g jar pickled red cabbage

HOW TO MAKE:

- Preheat the oven to 220°c. Boil a bowl of water and then simmer the potatoes for 5 minutes, then drain and put aside.
- In a huge ovenproof skillet, heat 1 tablespoon of oil in a large, on high heat and fry the bacon for 5 minutes until crispy. Add the carrots, onions, courgettes, onions, and garlic; season and then cook for 5 mins. Put pan in oven and bake for 25 to 30 mins before the veg is tender and gold.
- Meanwhile, heat the remaining oil into a skillet on medium-high heating and fry the eggs 2 to 3 mins or until cooked to your liking.
- Split the hash between two plates and top each with lettuce. Sprinkle with parsley and simmer, then serve with the pickled red cabbage onto both

Bacon and egg fried rice

Ingredients

- 350g long-grain rice, well rinsed
- 1 ½ tablespoon olive oil
- 100g streaky bacon, diced
- 2 peppers, finely chopped
- 2 red onions, finely chopped
- 200g carrots, peeled and coarsely grated
- 2 garlic cloves, crushed
- 5cm slice ginger, peeled and grated
- 1 red chili, finely chopped (optional)
- 2 eggs
- 2 teaspoon soy sauce

HOW TO MAKE

- Cook the rice in a big bowl of warm water for 10 mins until not quite tender. Drain, rinse with warm water and drain. Set aside.
- Meanwhile, warm ½ tablespoon oil in a skillet on a high heat and fry the

bacon for 5 to 7 minutes until golden and crispy. Remove from the pan using a slotted spoon and place aside. Add 1 tablespoon oil and fry the peppers for 10 minutes until lightly bubbling. Add the carrots, onions, ginger, garlic, and chili and fry over a moderate-high temperature for 5 mins more.

- Add the rice and bacon and simmer for 5 mins, stirring often. Push the rice mix to a single side of this pan and then crack the eggs to the gap. Beat the eggs with a wooden spoon, and then stir throughout the rice. Cook for 2 mins, then add the soy sauce and remove from heat. Split between 4 shallow bowls to serve.

Super-speedy prawn risotto

Ingredients:

- 100g diced onion
- 2 x 250g packs whole grain rice & quinoa

- 200g frozen garden peas
- 2 x 150g packs cooked and peeled king prawns
- 1/285g tote water-cress

SNACKS & DESSERTS RECIPES

Snow-flakes

Ingredients

- Won ton wrappers
- Oil
- Powdered -sugar

HOW TO MAKE:

- Cut won ton wrappers just like a snow-flake
- Heat oil. When hot, add won-ton, fry for approximately 30 seconds then flip over.
- Drain and add powdered sugar.

Lemon ricotta cookies with lemon glaze

Ingredients

- Two ½ cups all-purpose flour
- 1 teaspoon baking powder
- 1 teaspoon salt
- 1 tablespoon unsalted butter softened
- 2 cups of sugar
- 2 eggs
- 1 teaspoon (15-ounce) whole-milk ricotta cheese
- 3 tablespoon lemon juice
- 1 lemon

Glaze:

- ½ cups powdered sugar
- 3 tablespoon lemon juice
- 1 lemon

HOW TO MAKE:

- Preheat the oven to 375°F.

- Using a medium bowl combine the flour, baking powder, and salt. Set aside.
- From the big bowl blend the butter and the sugar levels. Beat sugar and butter with an electric mixer until and light for about three minutes. Add the eggs1 at a time and beating until fully mixed.
- Add the ricotta cheese, lemon juice, and lemon zest. Beat to blend. Stir in the dry ingredients.
- Line two baking sheets with parchment paper. Spoon the dough (approximately 2 tablespoons of each cookie) on the baking sheets. Bake for fifteen minutes, until slightly golden at the borders. Remove biscuits from the oven and let them stay in baking sheet for about 20 minutes.

Glaze:

- Combine the powdered sugar lemon juice and lemon peel in a small bowl and then stir until smooth. Spoon approximately ½ teaspoon on each cookie and make use of the back of the spoon to lightly disperse. Allow glaze harden for approximately two hours.

Home-made marshmallow fluff

Ingredients

- ¾ cup sugar
- ½ cup light corn syrup
- ¼ cup water
- ⅛ teaspoon salt
- 3 egg whites
- ¼ teaspoon cream of tartar
- 1 teaspoon
- ½ teaspoon vanilla extract

HOW TO MAKE:

- In a little pan, mix together sugar, corn syrup, salt, and water. Attach a candy thermometer into the side of this pan, but make sure it does not touch the underside of the pan.

- Combine egg whites and cream of tartar. Begin to whip on medium speed with the whisk attachment.
- Meanwhile, turn a burner on top and place the pan with the sugar mix onto heat. Pour mix in to boil at 240°F, stirring periodically.
- The aim is to have the egg whites whipped to soft peaks and also the sugar heated to 240°F at the same moment. Simply stop stirring the egg whites once they hit soft peaks.
- Once the sugar is ready, turn heat to low. Insert a little quantity of the popular sugar mix. Insert another little sum of the sugar mix. Carry on adding mix slowly and that means you never scramble the egg whites.
- After all of the sugar is added into the egg whites, decrease the speed of the this mixer and also keep mixing concoction for around 7 to 9 minutes until the fluff remains glossy and stiff.

When it reaches 5 minutes add the vanilla extract.
- Use fluff immediately or store in an airtight container in the fridge.

Guilt totally free banana ice-cream

Serves 3

Ingredients

- 3 ripe banana - peeled and chopped
- A couple of chocolate chips
- Two tablespoon skim milk

HOW TO MAKE:

- Pour the ingredients into a food processor and blend until creamy.
- Freeze and appreciate afterward.

Perfect little PB snack balls

Ingredients

- ½ cup chunky peanut butter
- 3 tablespoon flax seeds

- 3 tablespoon wheat germ
- 1 tablespoon honey or agave
- ¼ cup powdered sugar

HOW TO MAKE:

- Blend dry ingredients and honey and peanut butter.
- Mix well and roll into chunks and then roll into wheat germ.

Dark chocolate pretzel cookies

Ingredients

- 1 cup yogurt
- ½ teaspoon baking soda
- ¼ teaspoon salt
- ¼ teaspoon cinnamon
- 4 tablespoon butter (softened)
- 1/3 cup brown sugar
- 1 egg
- ½ teaspoon vanilla
- ½ cup dark chocolate chips
- ½ cup pretzels, chopped

HOW TO MAKE:

- Preheat oven to 180°C.
- Mix together the sugar, butter, vanilla, and egg in a medium bowl.
- In another bowl, stir together the flour, baking soda, and salt.
- Stir the bread mixture in, using all the moist components, along with the chocolate chips and pretzels until just blended.
- Drop large spoonsful of dough on an unlined baking sheet.
- Let it bake for about 15 to 17 minutes, or until the bottoms are somewhat all crispy.
- Allow cooling on a wire rack.

Mascarpone cheesecake with almond crust

Ingredients

Crust:

- ½ cup slivered almonds

- 8 teaspoon cup graham cracker crumbs
- 2 tablespoon sugar
- 1 tablespoon salted butter melted

Filling:

- 1 (8-ounce) packages cream cheese, room temperature
- 1 (8-ounce) container mascarpone cheese, room temperature
- ¾ cup sugar
- 1 teaspoon fresh lemon juice
- 1 teaspoon vanilla extract
- 2 large eggs, room temperature

HOW TO MAKE:

Crust:

- Preheat oven to 180°C. You will need a 9-inch diameter round the pan.
- Finely grind the almonds, cracker crumbs and sugar into a food processor.

- Put in the butter and continue to process until it forms moist crumbs.
- The almond mixture should be pressed on the base of the prepared pan
- Bake the crust until its set and start to brown, about 1 to 2 minutes. Cool. Reduce the oven temperature to 325°F.

Filling:

- In a large bowl, beat the mascarpone cheese, cream cheese, and sugar until it becomes smooth, using an electric mixer. Occasionally scrape down the sides of the jar using a rubber spatula. Beat in the lemon juice and vanilla.
- Add1 egg one at a time, beating until combined after each addition.
- Pour the cheese mixture on the crust from the pan. Put the pan into a big skillet or Pyrex dish; pour enough hot water into the pan so that it is halfway up. Bake until the middle of this filling

moves slightly when the pan is gently shaken, for about 1 hour (the dessert will get hard when it's cold).

- Transfer the cake to a stand and cool for 1 hour. Refrigerate until the cheesecake is cold, for at least eight hours.

Topping:

- Squeeze just a small thick cream in the microwave using chopped dark chocolate. Afterward, get a ziploc baggie and cut out a hole at the corner, then pour the melted chocolate into the baggie and used to decorate the cake.

Marshmallow popcorn balls

Ingredients

- 2 bags of microwave popcorn
- 1 (12.6 ounces) m&m's
- 3 cups honey roasted peanuts

- 1 pkg. 16 ounce massive marshmallows
- 1 cup butter, cubed

HOW TO MAKE:

- In a bowl, blend the popcorn, peanuts and m&m's.
- In a big pot, combine marshmallows and butter.
- Cook using medium-low heat.
- Insert popcorn mix, blend thoroughly
- Spray muffin tins with non-stick cooking spray.
- When cool enough to handle, spray hands together with non-stick cooking spray and then shape into chunks and put into the muffin tin to carry shape.
- Add Popsicle stick into each chunk and then let cool.
- Wrap each serving in vinyl when chilled.

Home-made ice-cream drumsticks

Ingredients

- Vanilla ice cream
- Two Lindt hazelnut chunks
- Magical shell - out chocolate
- Sugar levels
- Nuts
- Parchment newspaper

HOW TO MAKE:

- Soften ice cream and mix topping
- Fill underside of sugar with magic and nuts shell and top with ice-cream.
- Wrap parchment paper around cone and then fill cone over about 1.5 inches across the top of the cone
- Sprinkle with magical nuts and shells.
- Freeze for about 20 minutes, before the ice cream is eaten.

Ultimate chocolate chip cookie n' Oreo fudge brownie bar

Ingredients

- 1 cup (2 sticks) butter, softened
- 1 cup granulated sugar
- ¾ cup light brown sugar
- Two large egg
- 1 tablespoon pure vanilla extract
- Two 2 ½ cups all-purpose flour
- 1 teaspoon baking soda
- 1 teaspoon lemon
- 2 cups (12 oz) milk chocolate chips
- 1 package double stuffed Oreos
- 1 family-size (9×1 3) brownie mixture
- ¼ cup hot fudge topping

HOW TO MAKE:

- Preheat oven to 180°C.
- Mix the butter and sugars in a large bowl using an electric mixer, at medium speed for 35 minutes.

- Put in the vanilla and eggs and mix thoroughly combine. In another bowl, whisk together the flour, baking soda and salt, and slowly incorporate in the mixer until everything is combined.
- Stir in chocolate chips.
- Spread the cookie dough at the bottom of a 9×13 baking dish that is wrapped with wax paper and then coat with cooking spray.
- Shirt with a coating of Oreos. Add in brownie mix, adding an optional ¼ cup of hot fudge directly into the mixture.
- Stir the brownie batter within the cookie-dough and Oreos.
- Use a foil to cover and bake at 180°C for half an hour.
- Remove foil and continue baking for another 15 to 25 minutes.
- Let cool before cutting brownies.

Crunchy chocolate chip coconut macadamia nut cookies

Ingredients

- 1 cup yogurt
- ½ teaspoon baking soda
- ½ teaspoon salt
- 1 tablespoon of butter, softened
- 1 cup firmly packed brown sugar
- ½ cup sugar
- 1 large egg
- ½ cup semi-sweet chocolate chips
- ½ cup sweetened flaked coconut
- ½ cup coarsely chopped dry-roasted macadamia nuts
- ½ cup raisins

HOW TO MAKE:

- Preheat the oven to 325°F.
- In a little bowl, whisk together the flour, oats and baking soda and salt; then place aside.

- In your mixer bowl, mix together the butter/sugar/egg mix.
- Mix flour and oats until just combined and stir into the chocolate chips, raisins, nuts, and coconut.
- Place outsized bits on a parchment-lined cookie sheet.
- Bake for 1 to 3 minutes, before biscuits are only barely golden brown.
- Remove from the oven and then leave the cookie sheets to cool for at least 10 minutes.

Peach and blueberry pie

Ingredients

- 1 box of noodle dough

Filling:

- 5 peaches, peeled and chopped
- 3 cups strawberries
- ¾ cup sugar
- ¼ cup bread
- Juice of ½ lemon

- 1 egg yolk, beaten

HOW TO MAKE:

- Preheat oven to 400°F.
- Place dough in a 9-inch pie plate
- In a big bowl, combine tomatoes, sugar, bread, and lemon juice, then toss to combine. Pour into the pie plate, mounding at the center.
- Take some of the bread and cut into bits, then put in a pie skirt and put the dough in addition to pressing on edges.
- Brush crust with egg wash then sprinkles with sugar.
- Set onto a parchment paper-lined baking sheet.
- For approximately 20 minutes bake at 400°F, until crust is browned at borders.
- Turn oven down to 350, bake for another 40 minutes.
- Remove and let sit at least 30minutes.
- Have with vanilla ice-cream.

Pear, cranberry and chocolate crisp (dessert)

Ingredients

- Crumble topping
- ½ cup pasta flour
- ½ cup brown sugar
- 1 teaspoon cinnamon
- ⅛ teaspoon salt
- ¾ cup yogurt
- ¼ cup sliced peppers
- 1/3 cup butter, melted
- 1 teaspoon vanilla
- Filling
- 1 tablespoon brown sugar
- ¼ cup dried cranberries
- 1 teaspoon lemon juice
- Two handfuls of milk chocolate chips

HOW TO MAKE:

- Preheat oven to 375.
- Spray a casserole dish with a butter spray.

- Put all of the topping ingredients - flour, sugar, cinnamon, salt, nuts, legumes
- Add butter into a bowl and then mix. Set aside.
- In a large bowl combine the sugar, lemon juice, pears, and cranberries.
- Once fully blended move to the prepared baking dish.
- Spread the topping evenly over the fruit.
- Bake for about half an hour.
- Spread chocolate chips out at the top.
- Cook for another 10 minutes.
- Drink or have with ice cream.

Apricot oatmeal cookies

Ingredients

- ½ cup (1 stick) butter, softened
- 2/3 cup light brown sugar packed
- 1 egg
- ¾ cup all-purpose flour
- ½ teaspoon baking soda

- ½ teaspoon vanilla extract
- ½ teaspoon cinnamon
- ¼ teaspoon salt
- ½ cups chopped oats
- ¾ cup yolks
- ¼ cup sliced apricots
- 1/3 cup slivered almonds

HOW TO MAKE:

- Preheat oven to 180°C.
- In a big bowl combine with the butter, sugar, and egg until smooth.
- In another bowl whisk the flour, cinnamon, baking soda, and salt all together.
- Mix the ingredients into the bowl with the butter and sugar.
- Now stir in almonds, oats, raisins, and apricots.
- In this time, it's much better to cool dough (therefore, your biscuits are thicker)

- Scoop biscuits into some parchment-lined (easier removal and wash up) cookie sheet - around two inches apart.

Chapter 7
21 DAY MEAL-PLAN

Day 1

Breakfast:

- Morning meal egg muffins
- or chickpea flour omelette muffins
- Oatmeal (peanut buttercup)
- Snack: banana slices and peanut butter

Lunch:

- Chicken salad
- or easy broccoli salad (almond lemon dressing)
- Snack: cucumber (half) with two tablespoons hummus

Dinner:

- Garlic shrimp in coconut coffee, tomatoes and cilantro zucchini, pea and spinach pesto risotto

Day 2

Breakfast:

- Leftover egg
- or chick-pea muffins
- or peanut buttercup oatmeal
- Snack: apple with sunflower seed/pumpkin seed course combination

Lunch:

- Garlic shrimp in coconut milk, cilantro and tomatoes
- or left-over zucchini, pea and spinach pesto risotto
- Snack: celery sticks with guacamole

Dinner:

- Taco salad
- or wild rice burrito bowl with cilantro-lime avocado dressing

Day 3

Breakfast:

- Egg and vegetable basil (scrambled)
- or cheesy tofu (scrambled)
- Snack: celery sticks together with peanut butter and raisins

Lunch:

- Taco salad
- or rice (wild) burrito bowl
- Snack: hard boiled eggs and orange
- or a couple of roasted chickpeas

Dinner:

- Turkey, kale along with cauliflower soup
- or navy bean soup with crispy kale

Day 4

Breakfast:

- Cranberry pecan overnight oats
- Snack: cucumber pieces with hummus

Lunch:

- Avocado tuna salad
- or shredded tofu pesto sandwich
- Snack: apple pieces sprinkled with cinnamon and almonds

Dinner:

- Leftover turkey, kale and cauliflower soup
- or navy bean soup with crispy kale

Day 5

Breakfast:

- Protein pancakes
- or paleo vegan pancakes
- Snack: pear and pistachios

Lunch:

- Orange almond salad using avocado
- or fall harvest salad with pomegranate vinaigrette
- Snack: skinny pop popcorn along with hardboiled egg

Dinner:

- Seafood zucchini pasta
- or avocado pesto zucchini noodles

Day 6

Breakfast:

- Leftovers reheated protein
- or vegan pancakes
- Snack: banana slices with peanut butter

Lunch:

- Leftover seafood zucchini pasta
- or avocado pesto zucchini noodles

- Snack: baby carrots along with guacamole

Dinner:

- Hearty bean chowder

Day 7

Breakfast:

- Grain-free pumpkinseed breakfast cereal
- Snack: pear and almonds

Lunch:

- Leftover hearty bean chowder
- Snack: corn thin cakes served with guacamole and fresh salsa

Dinner:

- Chicken (orange) using simple salad
- or orange tofu

Day 8

Breakfast:

- 5-minutes flourless chocolate banana zucchini muffins
- or pumpkin blueberry muffins
- Snack: brown rice salad, peanut butter, and a spoonful of honey or maple syrup

Lunch:

- Leftover orange poultry with salad
- Vegan: Orange tofu
- Snack: small tomatoes tossed with black beans and avocado

Dinner:

- Darkened steak with mango avocado salsa
- or smoky tempeh using fresh peach and cherry tomato salsa

Day 9

Breakfast:

- Blueberry pistachio apple sandwiches
- Snack: 5-minutes flourless chocolate banana zucchini muffins

Lunch:

- Leftover grilled salmon with mango salsa
- or smoky tempeh
- Snack: corn thins along with guacamole

Dinner:

- Jalapeno turkey burgers
- or spicy vegan Portobello mushroom burgers

Day 10

Breakfast:

- Morning meal egg muffins

- or crust
- Snack: baked sweet potato with banana, cinnamon and peanut butter

Lunch:

- Cauliflower bowls
- Snack: Chickpeas (roasted) and berries

Dinner:

- Leftover cauliflower mushroom bowl using jalapeno turkey burgers
- or spicy vegan Portobello mushroom burger

Day 11

Breakfast:

- Blueberry pistachio apple sandwiches
- Snack: raspberries and pistachios

Lunch:

- Avocado chicken Waldorf salad
- or vegan Waldorf salad

- Snack: left-over cherry egg yolks
- or vegan egg yolks

Dinner:

- Sweet potato noodles with almond dijon vinaigrette

Day 12

Breakfast:

- Leftover breakfast egg yolks
- or vegan egg yolks
- Snack: banana pieces with vanilla butter and dusted with cocoa powder

Lunch:

- Leftover sweet potato noodles
- Snack: baby carrots and hummus

Dinner:

- Shrimp and asparagus stir fry
- or sweet and sour tofu

Day 13

Breakfast:

- Sweet potato toast
- Snack: inch one Lara bar

Lunch:

- Avocado and shrimp salad (utilizing leftover beans)
- or sweet-sour and sweet tofu
- Snack: skinny pop popcorn along with hardboiled egg
- or couple of roasted chickpeas

Dinner:

- Roasted garlic and herb cod
- or easy roasted veggie pizza bites

Day 14

Breakfast:

- Sweet potato toast
- Snack: cucumber pieces and hummus

Lunch:

- Leftover roasted herb and garlic cod
- Snack: larabar

Dinner:

- Sheet pan chili lime shrimp fajitas
- or one-pan Mexican quinoa

Day 15

Breakfast:

- Berries, beef and coconut shreds cereal
- Snack: dried, pitted dates along with peanut-butter

Lunch:

- citrus chicken strips over a spinach salad
- Snack: hard-boiled eggs
- or couple roasted chickpeas and carrots with hummus

Dinner:

- tomato basil soup

Day 16

Breakfast:

- Apple spice overnight oats
- Snack: brown rice with peanut butter and banana pieces

Lunch:

- Leftover tomato noodle soup
- Snack: raw pepper strips together with hummus and pumpkin

Dinner:

- Harvest chicken salad
- or lentil cucumber salad

Day 17

Breakfast:

- Leftover apple spice overnight oats

- Snack: dried pieces of bread and dates

Lunch:

- Leftover harvest chicken salad
- or lentil cucumber salad
- Snack: apple and couple roasted chickpeas

Dinner:

- steak and veggie quinoa casserole
- or vegan Shepard's pie with gravy

Day 18

Breakfast:

- Fresh fruit and rice breakfast pudding
- Snack: banana and pistachios

Lunch:

- Greek quinoa salad
- Snack: chocolate cherry energy bites

Dinner:

- Leftover chicken and veggie quinoa casserole

Day 19

Breakfast:

- Black bean scramble
- or spiced chickpea breakfast scramble
- Snack: chocolate cherry energy bites

Lunch:

- Leftover green quinoa salad
- Snack: Walnuts and 100 percent apple chips

Dinner:

- Chicken noodle soup (homemade)
- or curried lentils butternut squash soup

Day 20

For Breakfast:

- Banana oat protein muffins
- Snack: apple chips (dipped in peanut butter)

Lunch:

- Homemade chicken noodle soup
- or curried butternut squash soup
- Snack: chocolate cherry energy bites

Dinner:

- Steak fajita nachos (I propose having "Mary's gone crackers" rather than creating homemade bread):

Day 21

Breakfast:

- Leftover banana oat protein muffins snack
- or chewy lemon oatmeal bites

Lunch:

- cashew tuna salad cucumber bites (utilize a vegan mayo)
- or simple chickpea salad with tomato
- Snack: baby tomatoes and pineapple slices tossed in olive oil, balsamic vinegar plus a pinch of pepper

Dinner:

- Grilled chicken and veggie bowls (make 8 servings to serve for 1week)
- or chick-pea taco Buddha bowl

References

1. Goggins, A., and Matten, G. (2018). "The Sirtfood Diet." Gallery Books.
2. https://www.abbeyskitchen.com/the-sirtfood-diet/
3. https://www.womenshealthmag.com/weight-loss/a19962137/sirtfood-diet-can-it-help-you-lose-weight/
4. https://www.health.harvard.edu/staying-healthy/calorie-counting-made-easy
5. https://www.healthline.com/nutrition/do-low-fat-diets-work#heart-disease
6. https://www.ncbi.nlm.nih.gov/pubmed/22208554
7. https://www.besthealthmag.ca/best-eats/nutrition/15-foods-to-eat-for-glowing-skin-and-healthy-hair/
8. https://health.gov/dietaryguidelines/2015/

9. https://www.hhs.gov/fitness/eat-healthy/dietary-guidelines-for-americans/index.html
10. https://lpi.oregonstate.edu/mic/food-beverages/glycemic-index-glycemic-load
11. https://www.pomona.edu/administration/dining/health-wellness/macronutrients
12. https://www.hsph.harvard.edu/nutritionsource/what-should-you-eat/protein/
13. https://www.google.com/amp/s/www.delish.com/food-news/amp30752844/what-is-sirtfood-diet/
14. https://www.healthline.com/nutrition/sirtfood-diet#section5
15. https://sirtfooddiet.net/articles/capers-powerful-sirtfood/
16. https://www.brunet.ca/en/health/health-tips/9-food-combinations-that-offer-incredible-health-benefits/

Lightning Source UK Ltd.
Milton Keynes UK
UKHW020831151220
375245UK00004B/829

9 781801 144209

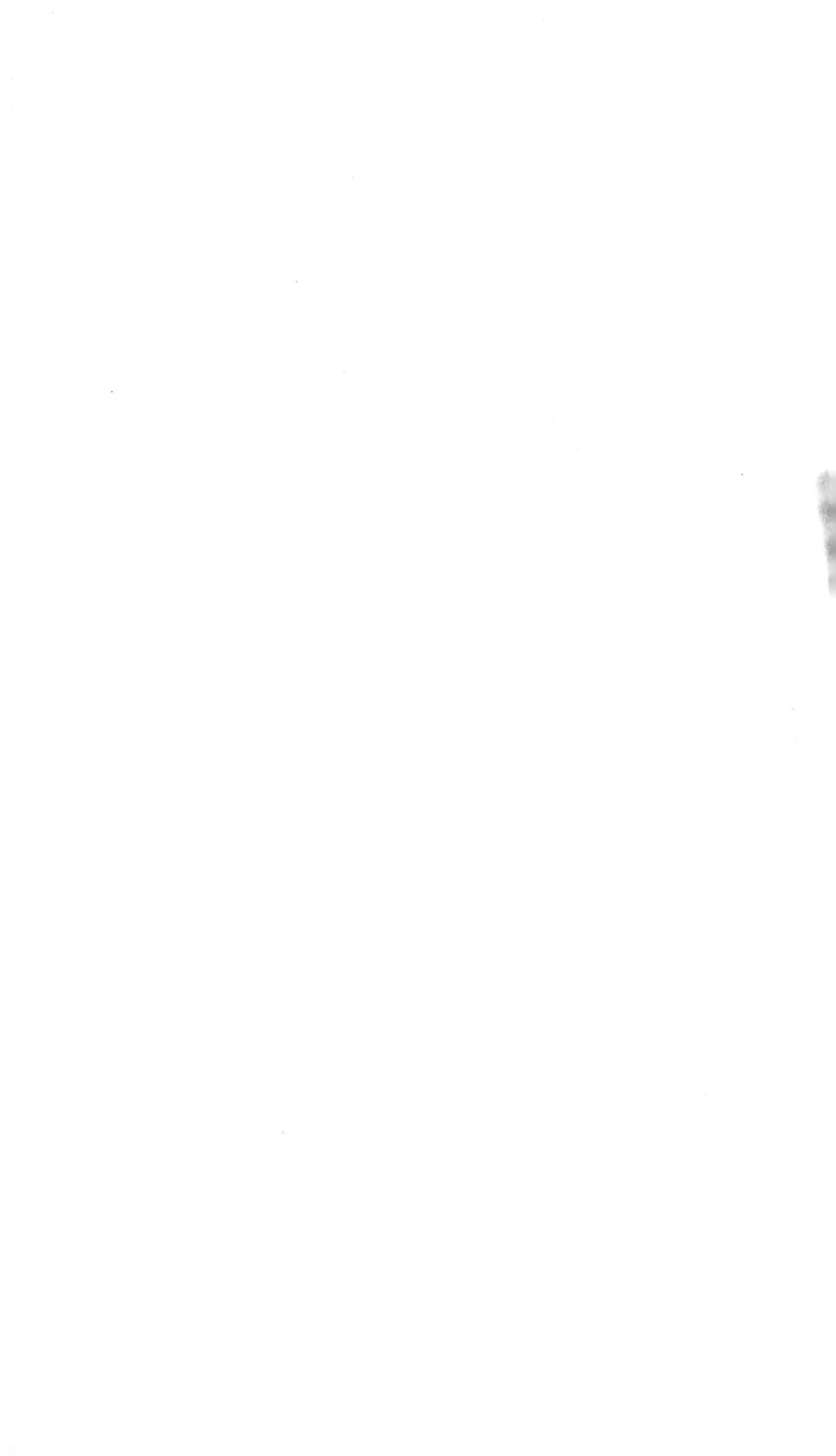